# DIET EARTH

# DIET EARTH

## The Conant Method: The True Nutritional Solution

Daryl Conant, M.Ed

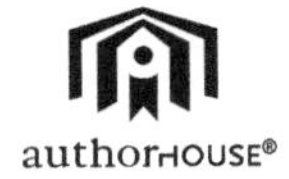

authorHOUSE®

*AuthorHouse™*
*1663 Liberty Drive*
*Bloomington, IN 47403*
*www.authorhouse.com*
*Phone: 1-800-839-8640*



*First published by AuthorHouse 10/30/2010*

*ISBN: 978-1-4520-1438-8 (e)*
*ISBN: 978-1-4520-1437-1 (sc)*

*Library of Congress Control Number: 2010905371*

*Printed in the United States of America*

*This book is printed on acid-free paper.*

# Table of Contents

# Dedication

I would like to dedicate this book to my family: Joy, Perrin, Avery and Faith. Thank you for your support and patience through this project, I love you all very much. I would also like to dedicate this book to my good friend Ron Kosloff, whose inspiration and guidance over the years have motivated me to write this book. Thank you.

Thank you Bob, Loryn, and Will for all your help.

Finally, I would like to dedicate this book to all my friends who support The Fitness Nut House™ in Kennebunk, Maine. Thank you all for your loyalty as it truly means everything to me. Small businesses are the backbone of America.

Diet EARTH has been written for anyone who wishes to add good nutrition and exercise into their personal and professional lives. Readers will learn that part of proper nutrition is being aware of the poisons in the foods that we eat and understanding how to avoid them. They will also learn about what exercise can do for the body, mind and spirit. A program of sensible, healthful eating and regular exercise does not mean rigorous dieting and extreme fatigue. The training and nutrition practices I describe throughout this book I like to call the "Conant Method: The True Nutritional Solution." A well-fed body that is sensibly and routinely exercised will give you the kind of body that will provide the stamina you need for times of physical and emotional stress. My final six words are "wait no longer, feel better today."

*--Daryl Conant, M.Ed*

*I can do all things through Christ who strengthens me.*
*Phil. 4:13*

## Disclaimer

The information provided in this book is not intended to treat, diagnose, or cure illness or disease. Check with your primary care physician before changing or starting a new nutrition plan based on the information in this book.

*Third Edition: October 2010*

# Preface

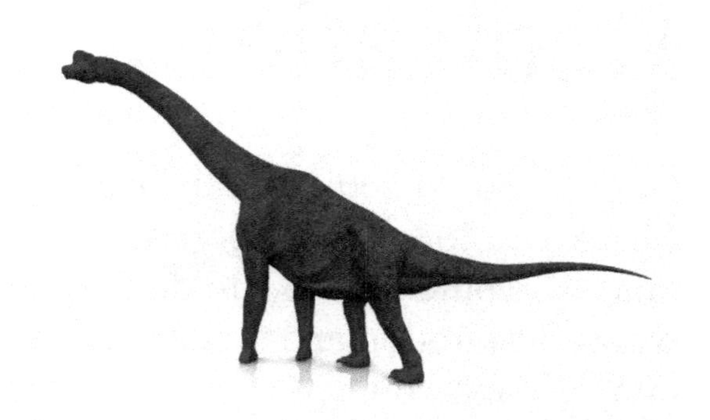

Earth is a living, breathing organism. The survival of Earth is dependent on the care and respect human beings have for it. Once the Earth decides its time for a change it will destroy its outer surface and regenerate a newer, cleaner environment. Human beings feel that they have the power to control the events that occur in the Earth's atmosphere. This is foolish! I believe the Earth is designed to cleanse itself when the atmosphere reaches toxic levels. We have evidence of this happening in the past. Thousands of years ago the Earth had primitive inhabitants. The Earth was hot and full of vegetation and large dinosaurs. Man was not at the top of the food chain. There were volcanos spewing vast amounts of poisonous gases into the atmosphere. When the toxicity reached a dangerous level, the Earth transformed itself into a colder unit, forming what has been called the *ice age*. During the ice age, the dinosaurs died off. There was not enough vegetation for the dinosaurs to survive. Humans survived because they ate mostly protein.

The Earth destroyed the effects of what was happening on the outer shell of itself. Today, years later, we once again are faced with toxic pollution and the changing of the Earth's atmosphere. Perhaps we are headed into another ice age. Today, the polar ice caps are melting off at a faster rate than normal. This is a a residual effect of the last ice age. Scientists and the general public think that they can stop the melting of the ice polar caps. We can not! The polar ice caps have been melting for years. I believe that when the Earth's outer temperature gets too hot, then it will resort to another ice age cycle. We are ignorant to think that we are more powerful than the Earth. The Earth is the most powerful entity we know. Without all the natural resources the Earth provides we would no longer be living on this mysterious planet. Too many people take their life for granted and just assume that they will wake up tomorrow to continue doing the same old thing day in and day out. They do not see the miracle that it takes to breathe one breath at a time and enjoy the wonder of what the Earth offers.

Along with all the pollution infiltrating into our natural resources, our natural food supply is becoming depleted of vital nutrients. The cancer, diseases, and illnesses, that we are seeing and hearing about every day are increasing among Americans. You would think that with all the research that has been done over the past eighty years there would be a cure for cancer. However, a cure has not been found. I believe that the reason for so much disease and illness in our culture is because of the destruction of our natural food sources. Scientists cannot find a cure for cancer because there are so many different types of reactions from all the poisons and toxins that food companies are pumping into our bodies. We are fighting an uphill battle. If some of the money used on cancer research was used to research how our food is getting contaminated, I feel that many cancers and illnesses would be prevented.

Think about this for a moment. If we lived in a world free of toxins, pesticides, chemicals, and acid rain, illness and disease wouldn't be so prevalent. The earth was once pure and rich in nutrients. Not anymore. Today we are in a situation where the earth is being depleted of essential nutrients needed for all its inhabitants. We are slowly killing the Earth and those that live on it. The purpose of this book is to open your mind to the connection between human existence and the Earth's vital nutrient supply. The Earth can live without us but we cannot live without the Earth. The irony is that the Earth is composed of approximately seventy percent salt water. Yet, we are running out of drinkable water. It is projected that within two hundred years the Earth's water supply will be completely depleted. Hopefully, there will be some type of reverse-osmosis system that can change salt water into fresh drinking water. My concern for the people on Earth today is that they are not taking care of themselves in a manner that is propelling humans into more conscious beings. I feel that the human body is the greatest gift from God. There is so much more we need to learn as a species. Yet, we are stuck in a primitive operating system that has taken a step backwards in collective intelligence.

Nutrition is a complex science. There is no right or wrong answer. It is all about one's own bio-individuality. All I can do is give recommendations and to share what I believe to be the correct methods on how to nourish the body.

I encourage you to read this book with an open mind and take what you need from it to help develop a healthy nutritional plan. This book is not a stereotypical nutrition book filled with recipes and diet schedules. The purpose of this book is to teach you how to eat correctly and learn ways to boost your energy based on human physiology. Bon appétit!

# Energy The Basis of Life

Types of Energy

- Universal
- Vital (VNES)

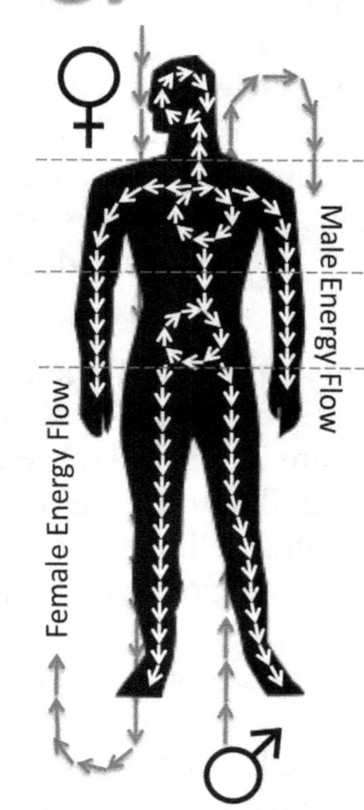


**Primary Energy**

Zone I: Nervous System

Zone II: Cardiorespiratory System

Zone III: Digestive System
Reproductive System (Female)

**Secondary Energy**

Zone IV: Reproductive System (Male)
(Female after Menopause)

Zone V: Skeletal Muscular System

♀ Female

♂ Male



All matter is made up of atoms. Atoms are comprised of three components: protons, electrons, and neutrons. The protons and the neutrons make up the center of the atom, which is called the nucleus, and the electrons fly around above the nucleus in a small cloud. Protons and electrons oppose each other, while neutrons remains neutral. Atoms do not make up energy. They do, however, produce energy due to the constant opposition of electrons and protons.

The human body is a temporary holding station for captured universal energy. Universal energy is the energy that cannot be seen. It is all of the atoms that make up the entire universe.

Human reproduction requires a male sperm cell and a female egg. Life begins with an electrical charge of energy as the sperm embeds into the egg. The atoms produce energy that begins to form molecules, which form cells. Cells multiply at a fast rate forming the embryo. The energy is captured in the heart where it will be the driving force of human life. Eventually the embryo becomes a fetus as more cells develop. After nine months a human baby is born.

Once the baby is out of the womb the cellular reproductive energy remains high. The vital organs, skin, bone and muscle are produced at a fast pace. Once the body reaches its peak development, around 23 to 24 years, the energy stabilizes. This energy can remain active as long as the body's energy zones are not compromised. When one or more of the energy zones are imbalanced, poor health can develop.

I have classified the body into two energy zones: *primary* and *secondary*. The primary energy zone consists of the nervous system, cardiorespiratory system, reproductive system (female) and the digestive system. The secondary energy zone consists of the muscular system and reproductive system (male).

The primary energy source is the energy that is involuntary. It is the energy that controls the vital nutrient exchange system (VNES). The vital nutrient exchange system is comprised of the vital organs that sustain human life. The brain, heart, kidneys, intestines, stomach, and liver are all part of the VNES. They are known as vital because without any one of these organs, the body cannot survive.

The nervous system, (Zone 1), is the electrical system of the body. Nerves deliver impulses to cells to elicit a reaction. This system is crucial to the function of human life. The brain and spine are vital components of the nervous system. The cardiorespiratory system, (Zone 2), is comprised of the heart, arteries, veins and lungs. It is important for delivering blood,oxygen, and vital nutrients to all the cells of the body. The heart is the master organ of the body. It is the main housing source of electrical conductivity. Keeping the heart healthy keeps the electrical conductivity strong.

The reproductive system and digestive system, Zone 3, are high-energy areas. The reproductive system for females requires increased levels of energy to help with the production of the egg each month. The menstrual cycle is an involuntary process that lasts between 30-40 years for females. For this reason I classify the reproductive system of a female as part of the primary energy zone. Though the female reproductive system is not necessary for survival, it is required to produce life.

The digestive system is important for nutrient exchange and elimination of wastes. There are two areas that are most dense with nerves: the spinal system and the digestive system. A lot of energy is required to operate the digestive system. If energy in the digestive system is compromised, the body is susceptible to illness, disease or even death. I have classified it as one of the primary energy zones.

The secondary energy source is the energy that is voluntary--we control the output. The secondary energy zone consists of the reproductive system (Zone IV) and skeletal muscular system (Zone V). The muscular system consists of skeletal muscle. Skeletal muscle has the potential capacity of producing large amounts of energy in the form of adenosine triphosphate (ATP). ATP is a high-energy phosphate compound that is produced in the mitochondria of cells and provides the body with energy. Muscle cells can produce high levels of ATP if they are being used. Thus to get the greatest benefit of ATP it is necessary to exercise to increase ATP's production. Dormant muscle cells produce little ATP, making energy production poor.

The reproductive system in males is a voluntary energy system. Though minimal amounts of VNES energy is used to help stimulate the production of sperm, the need is not life threatening. Therefore, the male reproductive system is not considered a primary energy source. Energy is driven to the area when stimulation of the male genitalia occurs. If energy production is poor then there will not be enough blood to pump into this area for proper functioning.

Females who have been through menopause fall into Zone IV of the secondary energy source, because their reproductive system has shut down production of the egg and is no longer in need of VNES energy. The female genitalia can be voluntarily stimulated to increase energy production.

The primary energy source is important for keeping the VNES healthy and running optimally. If there is an imbalance in any one of Zones 1-3, illness, disease and death can occur. Though it is not crucial for secondary energy sources to be activated daily, they do serve to boost energy by helping to make the primary energy sources more efficient.

All of the energy systems in all five zones work synergistically. If there is a blockage of energy in any one of these areas, especially in the primary energy sources, then good health is threatened. Blood pressure is one example of how a blocked energy zone can develop into disease. Poor dietary habits lead to a build up of fat around the visceral organs due to insufficient digestive processing. This excess fat can drain the body of VNES energy. Over time this can affect the heart and lung systems. High blood pressure develops, making the heart work harder to deliver oxygen throughout the body. Low levels of oxygen getting into the body will, over time, affect the brain. The brain has to have enough oxygen to function optimally. When it doesn't, parts of the brain can become dysfunctional.

Establishing good health within all the energy zones can help reduce the early onset of disease and provide for greater longevity.

Here are some ways to boost the energy systems of the body:

- Eating foods rich in nutrients
- Exercising
- Breathing (Meditation)

In this book, you will learn how to eat correctly and how to exercise effectively to boost the energy systems of your body. The objective of life is to live healthily and to improve longevity, to be able to enjoy every facet of the aging process. By keeping your primary energy source high you can have greater longevity. Exercising throughout all ages of life reinforces energy production in the body. Exercise forces blood to pump more strong throughout the body, which has been proven to strengthen the arteries, muscles, and bones, and improve cellular regeneration.

To understand how to take better care of yourself through proper nutrition and exercise practices it is important to know the genesis of nutrition.

# The Genesis of Nutrition

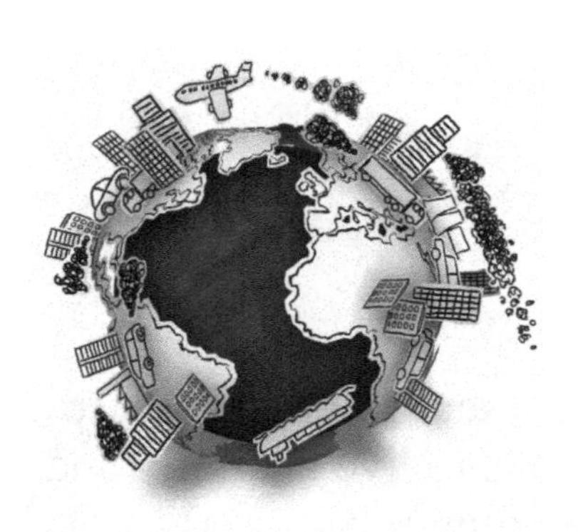

As long as Earth has existed, nutrition has been the driving force of life. Every living cell needs nutrients to survive. This is fundamental knowledge. Human nutrition began with primitive beings.

The earliest humans ate raw foods from the Earth. They most likely did not cook or prepare anything. They were primitive in nature and were instrumental in keeping the human gene pool alive. If nutrition was neglected during the earliest times of human life then I would not be writing this book because we would not exist. As primitive men became better hunters and gatherers they were able to hone in on what the body needed to survive--PROTEIN. Animal meat was the staple of primitive nutrition. Vegetation was secondary. If vegetables were the only source of food during this time of life, primitive man would not have survived. Protein is the most important aspect of human growth and development. Perhaps protein should be called "grow-tein" because of its importance in helping the body grow.

As mankind progressed into a more conscious and civilized being, nutrition was still centered on eating directly from the Earth. The foods from Earth were raw and densely rich in nutrients. Animal meat continued to be the staple of the diet. Farms became a way of life for most of the population. Families depended on the harvest for survival. Everyone in the family had a part in working the farm. The men hunted for meat, the children worked the land, gathered vegetables, milked the cows and goats, and women prepared the food to be consumed. The farm was a working entity and a way of survival. When the farm was in jeopardy, so was the family. Lack of food and nutrients resulted in disease and death. A human cannot live if he/she loses more than 60% of their body mass. Though a person can live many consecutive days without eating before dying, humans cannot live more than ten days without water. If the air temperature is in the range of 100 to 120 degrees fahrenheit, a person can only survive two days without water.

It has been established that human survival depends on eating the proper nutrients. Protein was and is the staple of the human diet. During the genesis of Earth there were no pollutants to degrade the nutrient-dense foods. It would be the industrial age that would change the composition of Earth's ecological system.

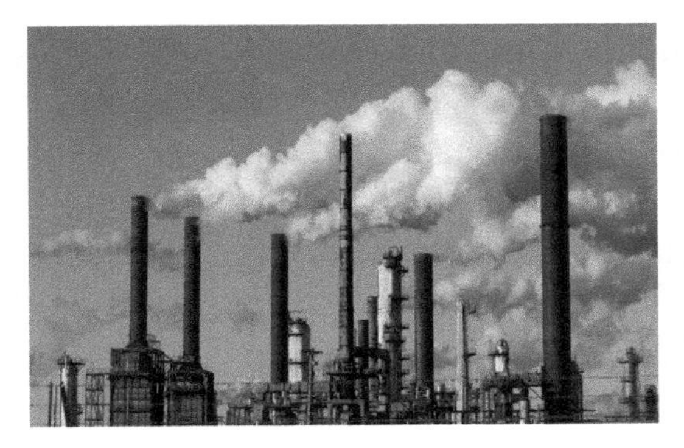

# The Industrial Age

The beginning of the destruction of the Earth's nutrient supply occurred when companies developed factories that emitted toxic pollution into the air. This pollution enters the atmosphere by mixing with clouds, causing acid rain. Acid rain falls to the Earth and covers everything. Acid rain gets into the water supply, plants, and animals. We eat these foods, and we ingest small amounts of toxic pollution into our bodies. Nothing can be done about this unless pollution is stopped. Even if the food is labeled organic, it is not entirely safe from acidic rain. All vegetables that are grown outdoors are affected by acid rain. Animals eat the grass that the rain has fallen on. We eat cows meat. Therefore, we consume agents from the acid rain. It is inescapable. We all ingest the agents of acid rain.

As the industrial age progressed, greater technology developed due to the increased growth of companies across the world. This expanse of technology led to great advances in transportation and communication. However, with the emergence of technology came the increase in human population.

Farms were still a way of life for most families in America. New inventions paved the way to helping the farms produce more food without having to rely solely on human labor. With an increase in the population, the need for food became more important. There is only so much food in the United States to sustain the population. If the food supply ever becomes compromised, then a problem develops because there would not be enough food for everyone. The natural food supply, which is food from natural resources and farms, became at risk during the industrial age.

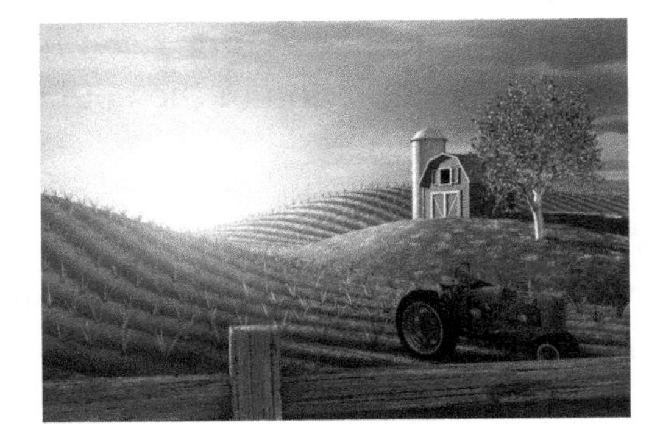

During the 1950's, the human reproductive rate was high, causing a surge in the population otherwise known as the Baby Boomer generation. This increase in population created a growing concern as to whether there was enough food to feed everyone. Men began working away from the home in manufacturing companies and factories. The family farm, which had been a staple of the family, began to decline in America.

Now that the farms began to produce less, the government had to devise new ways to help food last longer. The supply and demand of food was becoming a problem. Milk from farms would not last long in its raw state, so pasteurized milk became much more popular. Pasteurized and homogenized milk lasts four to six weeks without spoiling. Though this process was good for improving the longevity of milk, it eventually became a problem to human health.

As pasteurized milk became more popular among the masses so did food processing. Food processing is a way of extending the longevity of raw ingredients and transforming them into different compositions. Food processing helps to give greater marketability of food products and increases revenue for companies. Small farms cannot continue to provide enough real nutrition for the masses. If the country continues to depend solely on small family farms, then eventually the country will be overcrowded with people. With an overpopulated country and not enough natural food source the land will be depleted. This depletion in natural food will result in third-world conditions. Starvation and poor health will result.

Animal protein is essential for human growth and development. There are just too many people on Earth to live solely off of animal protein. In America, the number of slaughtered cows and chickens on a daily basis is very high. The government has had to regulate the production of slaughtered cattle, buffalo and chicken so that they wouldn't become extinct. If family farms continued to be the main provider of our society, then there wouldn't be enough animal protein to supply the masses.

To avoid the potential of having people living without food and having the country depleted of its natural food supply, processed food became the staple of the American diet.

From the mid 1900's to the present day, food processing has become big business. Most Americans eat processed food every day. Though processed food has helped reduce the depletion of the country's food supply, it has also contributed to the onset of disease.

Today, family-run farms are almost entirely extinct. The government now controls the agriculture of America. Commercial farmers produce huge crops to feed the masses. The technology of farm equipment has allowed farmers to keep up with the supply and demand of food. However, in order to protect the crops from insects and disease, farmers use pesticides. There doesn't seem to be much regulation on the release of pesticides used on the crops. Pesticides are poisons that kill off insects and reduce the diseases of grains, fruits, and vegetables. We ingest these foods and consume small amounts of the pesticides.

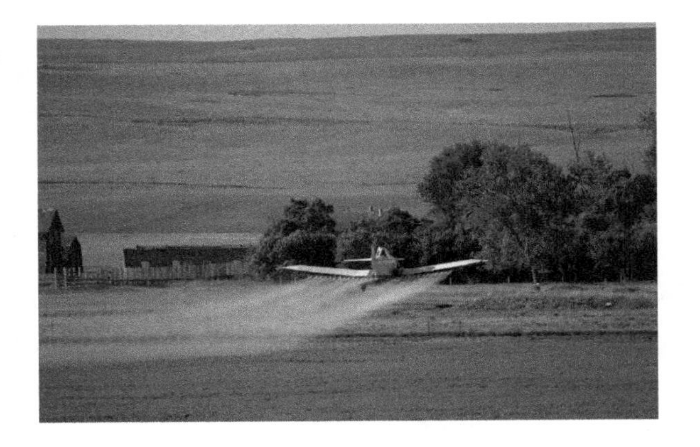

Throughout the centuries, the demand for natural food has increased. This increase in supply and demand has influenced the creation of food processing. True, natural food is hard to find nowadays. Ever since the end of family farms, the health of Americans has declined and the rise of disease and obesity has reached an all time high.

Diabetes was rarely heard of sixty years ago. Today, a person becomes diabetic every six seconds in America. Heart disease was not the number-one cause of death a hundred years ago; today it is. Colon, breast, prostate, esophageal, and skin cancers were small concerns fifty years ago. Now these cancers affect one out of every three people in America. It is no coincidence that right about the time family farms and true natural food went extinct that the rise in disease increased. Poor nutrition is directly related to all these diseases. Most diseases are nothing more than nutritional deficiencies. In America good nutrition is hard to come by. We all are subjected to ingesting poisons and pollutants. Eating organic food is better than eating non-organic food but, even organic foods have a certain number of toxins in them as a result of acid rain.

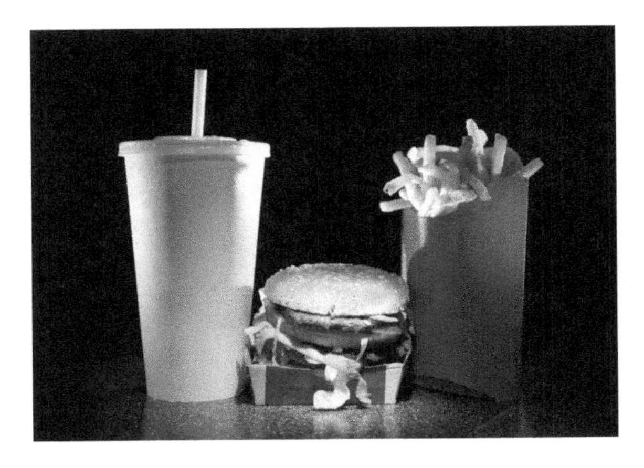

Eating a healthy diet full of organic foods and free-range meats is great for feeding the body. However, unless you have eaten like this all of your life, then you are still at risk of developing diseases related to toxins. Eating junk food filled with hydrogenated fats, soda, refined sugars and toxic preservatives throughout your life can cause disease even if you now eat only organic food.

# Processed Food

Processed foods contain many additives, preservatives, antibiotics, steroids, exocitotoxins, hydrogenated fats, and refined sugars. People seem to be concerned only with reading the label for calorie, protein, fat and sugar content. They seldom concern themselves with reading the ingredients for dangerous substances. Being ignorant about what you are eating could be the reason for illness or the early onset of disease. The following is an overview of some of the prevalent chemicals consumed every day by millions of Americans.

## *What's actually in our food?*

### Additives Preservatives

are substances added to food to preserve flavor or improve its taste and appeal. The following are examples:

- Blue 1 and 2
- Red 3
- Yellow 6
- Potassium Sorbate
- Benzoic Acid
- Sodium Benzoate
- Sucralose
- High Fructose Corn Syrup

**Blue 1 and 2**
An additive that gives color to foods. This has been linked to increasing brain tumors in lab rats.

Found commonly in:

- Candy
- Some ice cream
- Sodas
- Sports drinks

**Red 3**
Food coloring found in cherries (fruit cocktail) and in canned and baked goods. Found to cause thyroid tumors in lab rats. There is a high probability of this causing brain tumors in humans as well.

Found commonly in:
- Maraschino cherries
- Candy
- Some ice cream

**Yellow 6**
Third most-used food coloring. Has been found to cause adrenal gland and kidney tumors. It contains small amounts of carcinogens.

Found commonly in:
- Sausages
- Gelatin
- Baked goods
- Candy
- Many common foods

**Potassium Sorbate**
Prolongs food shelf life by protecting it against deterioration caused by microorganisms. Protects against fungi and yeast. Considered safe. Can cause allergic reactions in some people. This is considered rare.

Found commonly in:
- Many common foods
- Apple cider
- Dried meats
- Processed cheese

**Benzoic Acid**
Preservative that protects against fungi and yeast and prolongs shelf life. It has a sour taste and is potentially dangerous and cancer producing.

Found commonly in:
- Fruit juices
- Pickles
- Soft drinks

• Hummus dips

**Sodium Benzoate**
This is a preservative that protects against fungi and yeast and Prolongs shelf life. It is potentially dangerous and cancer producing.

Found commonly in:
• Salad dressings
• Condiments
• Soda
• Fruit juices
• Some processed foods
• Hummus dips

**Sucralose**
A sweetener that is 600 times sweeter than sucrose. It is used in small amounts to sweeten food products. It is safe if not over consumed. Sucralose is a chlorinated sugar that can cause headaches if over consumed. Low to moderate level intake is safe. Splenda is chlorinated sugar and is used as a sugar substitute. Splenda is dangerous if over-consumed.

Found commonly in:
• Canned drinks
• Candy
• Gum
• Sugar substitutes
• Diabetic foods
• Yogurts
• Pudding
• Ice cream
• Protein powders /bars /Drinks
• In foods labeled “diet” or “low calorie”

**High Fructose Corn Syrup**
This is a highly refined clear liquid derived from corn starch. It is a cheap way to sweeten food. It lasts longer on the shelf than sugar. HFCS contains a large amount of “free,” or unbound, fructose. Fructose (fruit sugar) in its normal form metabolizes in the liver before entering the blood stream. There is fiber in fructose that slows the absorption rate. HFCS can be easily manipulated to contain 80% fructose and 20% glucose. Glucose is the primary sugar that the body uses in all

metabolic processes. All sugar that enters the body must be converted to glucose before entering the bloodstream. The high content of fructose in HFCS poses a danger for the bloodstream. HFCS, when entering the bloodstream bypasses the insulin reactive receptor. This causes high concentrations of excess sugar to remain in the blood. Fat cells absorb the excess sugar. This can lead to obesity, heart disease, and high cholesterol levels. Eating HFCS is dangerous and should be avoided. Nothing good comes from HFCS.

Found commonly in:
- Most common foods
- Many junk foods
- Candy
- Cakes
- Pastries
- Packaged food
- Soda

**Stevia**
Known as a sweetleaf. A natural sweetener that has a long lasting sweet taste. It is a better alternative to artificial sweeteners (i.e. Splenda). This is a a safe sweetener and can be used in small amounts to provide a sweet taste to foods.

Found commonly in:
- A variety of organic food products

# Exocitotoxins

Exocitotoxins are the pathological process by which nerve cells are damaged and killed by glutamate and similar substances, which are commonly found in:

- Aspartame
- MSG: monosodium glutamate
- Acesulfame-K (Potassium)
- Sodium nitrate
- Hydrogenated vegetable oil

**Aspartame**

Aka Equal™, Nutrasweet™. This is a sweetener made from The methyl ester of a phenylalanine/aspartic acid dipeptide. This harmful substance has possible side effects if over-consumed such as: Cancer, diabetes, emotional disorders, menstrual problems, headaches, epilepsy/ seizures, and birth defects.

*Phenylalanine*: Too much of this substance excites the neurons in the brain to the point of cellular death. It is an isolated amino acid.

**MSG: Monosodium Glutamate**

This is a flavor enhancer with the following side effects: headaches, sweating, facial pressure, numbness, chest pain, nausea, rapid heart rate, sudden death, and sensitive neuron death.

Found commonly in

- Fast foods (Chinese)
- Salad dressings
- Meats
- Canned vegetables

**Sodium Nitrate**

This is an agent used as a preservative that forms agents known as nitrosamines that are cancer-producing in humans.

Found commonly in:

- Some non-organic beef jerky
- Cured meats
- Bacon/smoked meats
- Food Coloring and flavoring

**Acesulfame-K (Potassium)**
This is an artificial sweetener 200 times sweeter than sugar which has been found to cause cancer and affect the thyroid gland in animals.

Found commonly in:
- Baked goods
- Chewing gum
- Soft drinks

**Hydrogenated Vegetable Oil**
These are processed fats that produce tightly bound fat molecules, known as trans fats. HVO promotes the onset of heart disease and diabetes. HVO should be avoided at all costs.

Found commonly in:
- Margarine
- Vegetable shortening
- Crackers / cookies / baked goods / certain types of bread
- Salad dressing

People always tell me that eating junk foods in moderation is fine. They say " it's all about moderation." I disagree with this idea. I believe that moderation increases the risk of illness or disease. Here is something I have come up with to help you understand why eating junk foods in moderation is not good. There are two types of consumption factors when eating food: *acute and chronic.*

The ***Acute Consumption Factor*** is the immediate effect caused by eating a food. Once you eat the food, you get a head or stomach ache, or your pulse increases. Obviously this is not a desirable effect. Exocitotoxins produce an immediate effect once ingested; therefore, moderately eating these types of foods is not good.

The other consumption factor is the ***Chronic Consumption Factor***. This is eating foods that contain dangerous compounds in small amounts over a prolonged period of time. The ill effects do not immediately show up. They show up later on in life. A person who develops cancer or brain disease could potentially have been influenced by a toxic chemical early on in life, and their immune system has been fighting it throughout the years. One day the immune system can no longer defend against the toxic invader, and the toxins take over and become the dominant force in the body. This could be a result of chronic over-consuming of preservatives, additives, or exocitotoxins.

I strongly oppose the use of toxic chemicals to help preserve food. It is an unhealthy shame that eating real, natural food is becoming harder and harder to do. With all the technology and awareness we have about nutrition the United States cannot produce healthy, toxin-free foods to help nourish its people. Just look around at society and you will see millions of people who are sick, obese, diabetic and suffering from cancer, psychological disorders, and heart disease. I believe that the majority of these problems are related to ingesting toxic poisons throughout life.

It is interesting to me that people who are always trying to save money at the grocery store by purchasing the processed low-nutrient value foods are the ones who are always sick. Makes you wonder, doesn't it?

**There is a complete list in the appendix of preservatives, additives, and exocitotoxins. (Appendix I)**

# The Calorie Phenomenon

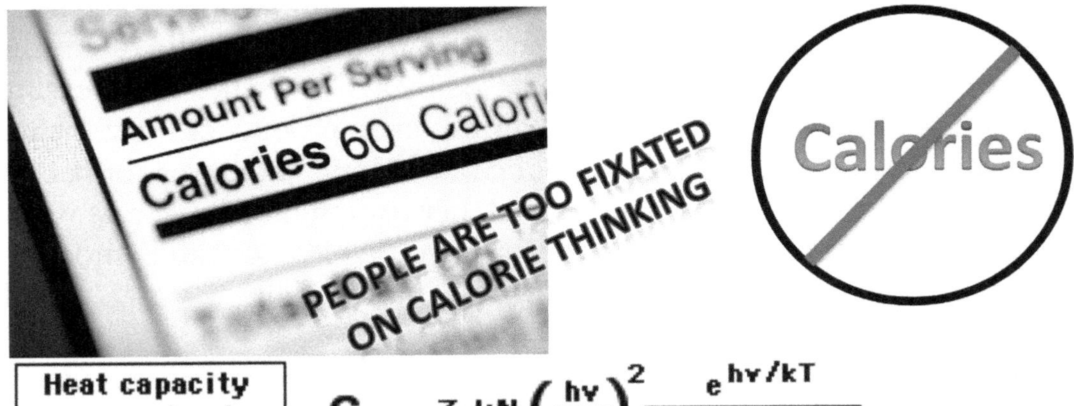


$$\text{Heat capacity per mole at constant volume} = C_v = 3\,kN\left(\frac{h\nu}{kT}\right)^2 \frac{e^{h\nu/kT}}{(e^{h\nu/kT}-1)^2}$$

where: T =absolute temperature; v = characteristic frequency; N = Avogadro's number
k = R/N = 1.380x10-15 erg/degree; and h = Planck's constant = 6.625 x 10-27 erg seconds**

Forms Of Heat Measurements:

Joules, Btu, calories, electron-volt, erg, watt hour, thermal, toe, Horse Power,

We are taught in our society that we must match our caloric intake with caloric expenditure. Though I agree with matching the heating effect of the body, I do not agree with consuming calories just for the sake of matching numbers with numbers. People are too fixated on calorie thinking.

A calorie is a measurement of heat. One calorie is equivalent to increasing the temperature of one gram of water one degree celsius. My question for you is to explain to me how a donut, made of nothing but garbage, can be 500 calories? Does this mean that a donut is increasing the heat of one gram of water one degree celsius just sitting on the shelf? It does not make sense to me. I have taken many courses in nutrition that all focused on calories. I believed in the calorie idea and even taught it to my clients for years. Then, one day, I just couldn't explain the calorie idea anymore. Here is when it changed for me.

I was doing a nutrition consultation with a woman and explaining the regular gibberish about caloric intake and expenditure. Then my client told me that she was taking the correct number of calories that I told her to take in. I had measured her resting metabolic rate earlier in the week. The resting metabolic rate is the product of expired gases (heat) that are released by active tissue. The measurement that it's tested in is calories. Remember, calories are a product of heat; the resting metabolic rate is heat. The resting metabolic rate caloric value was for her was measured at 1500 calories. I told her to match her resting metabolic rate with 1500 calories of food. And if she exercised then she would have to take in more calories, up to 1800, to keep from going into a caloric deficit.

She told me that she was taking in the right amount of calories to match her expenditure but she wasn't seeing a change in her body measurements, weight or appearance. In fact, she had gained five pounds. I asked her if she was following the balanced meal plan that I designed for her. She said that she could not eat all the food and decided to design her own meal plan. Although she matched the intake with 1500 calories, the types of food she chose were a far cry from what I had prescribed. Her argument was that I told her she needed 1500 calories and she

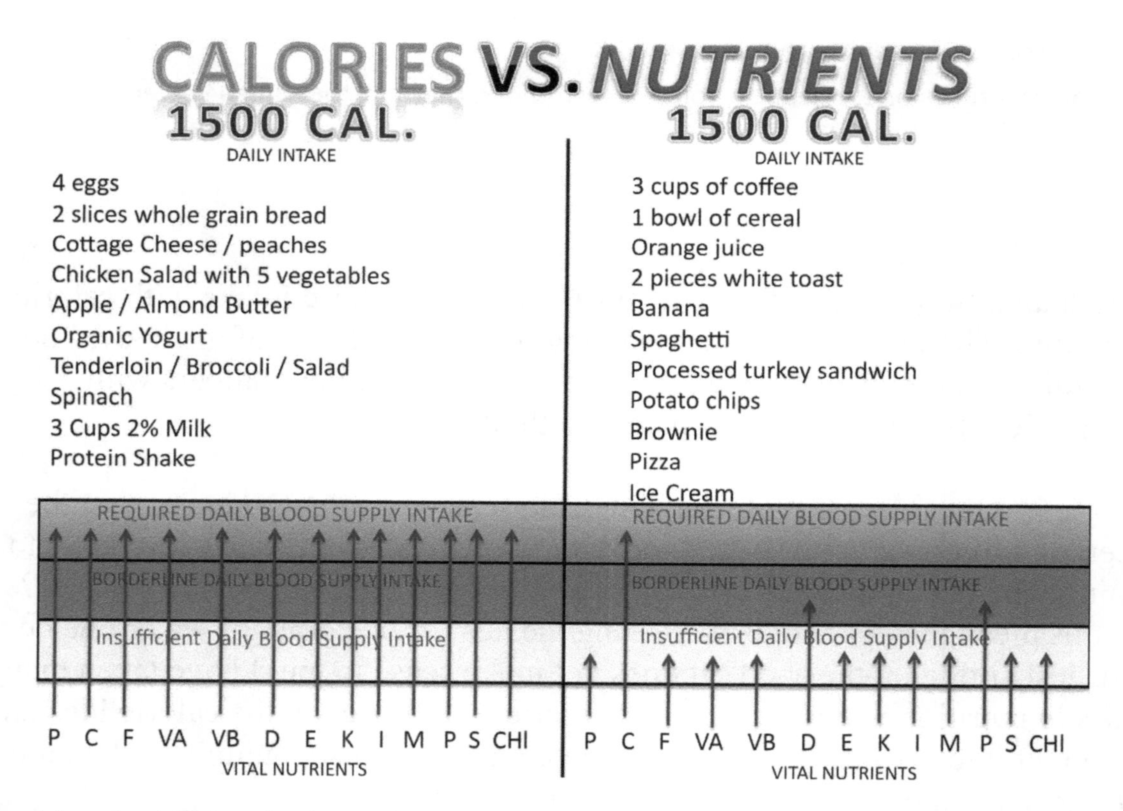


was taking in 1500 calories. The foods she took in were in the form of ice cream, pasta, and chips, all of which have very little useable healthy nutrients. So altogether she was correct in taking in 1500 calories, but she was totally incorrect in that she was not in taking the vital nutrients her body's VNES (vital nutrient exchange system) needed.

Suddenly my thought cycle shifted into a whole different realm. I began talking about ***vital nutrients***. Vital nutrients are the required vitamins, minerals, proteins, low glycemic carbohydrates, fats and water that the body needs. Vital nutrients feed the vital organs of the body. Vital organs are the organs that have to survive to sustain our heart, brain, lungs, kidneys, stomach liver, intestines--basically what we need for life. I explained to my client that she needed to fill her body up with vital nutrients and not worry about counting calories anymore. The reason why she couldn't eat all the food was because it was so nutrient-dense. Once the body is fed with the correct amount of nutrients, it will no longer activate the hunger response. Calories do not matter. How many vital nutrients you take in does.

**From that day on I never talked about calories again. Now I talk about my own theory of nutrition and one that makes sense to me. It is called Metabolic Nutrition.**

Here is another scenario. A girl was not eating enough food, and her doctor was concerned about her weight. He told her that she needed to eat more calories. He said, " I don't care what foods you eat, just as long as you take in more calories. You can eat cake, candy, and ice cream to help take in more calories." ARE YOU KIDDING ME? This is an actual medical doctor telling a teenage girl to eat junk food and that it didn't matter what it was as long as she got her caloric intake up. This is appalling to me. Not only is this wrong but it also influences the onset of eating disorders. Doctors should be prescribing proper nutrient intake to their patients, not calories.

Calorie thinking is an incorrect way to control eating. It is ignorant thinking. If someone can actually show me a calorie then maybe I will subscribe to calorie thinking. You can't see a calorie because they don't exist. A calorie is only a measurement of heat. Doctors misinterpret calories and food companies exploit calories as a way to sell more products.

# The Metabolic Wheel

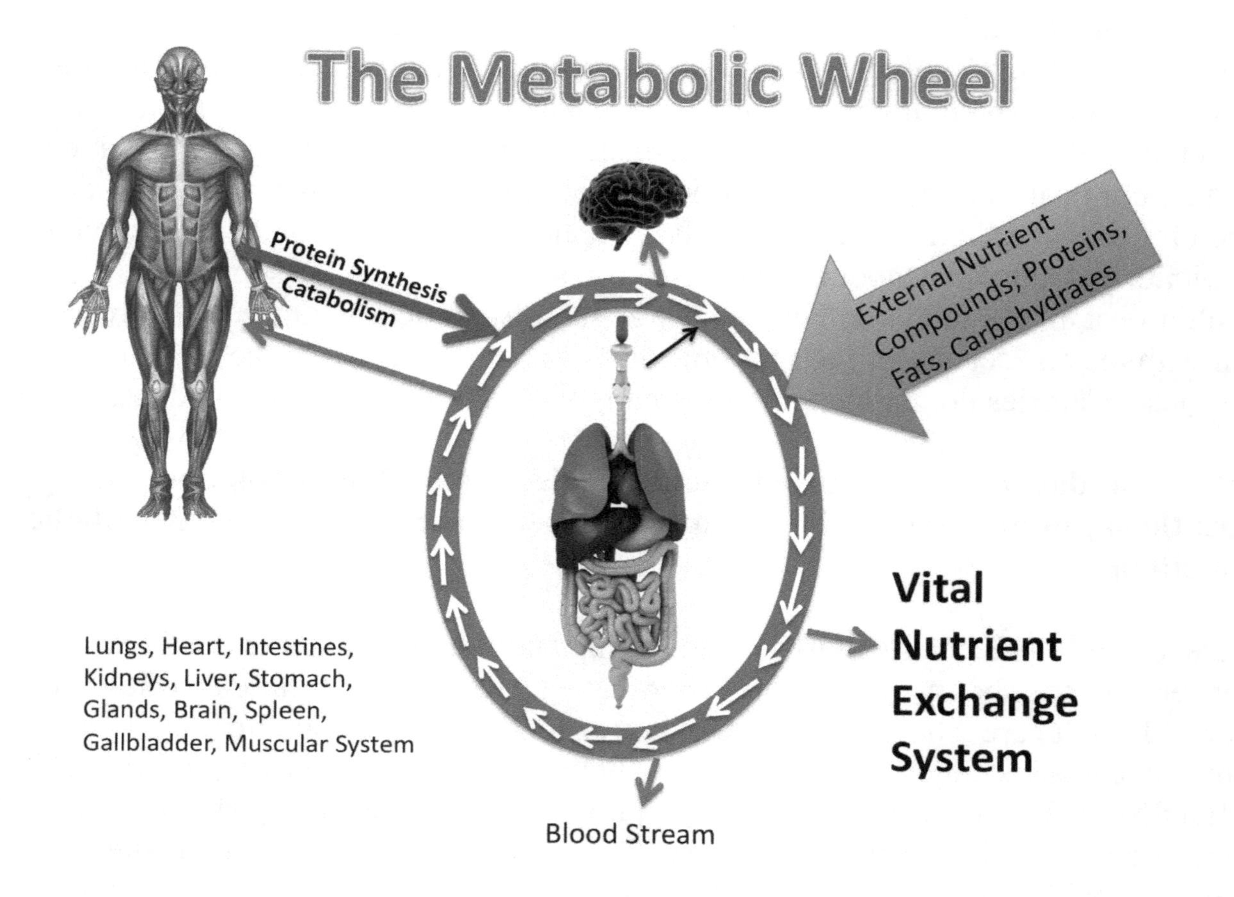


The metabolic wheel is a concept that I have come up with to help explain the complexity of protein, sugar and fat metabolism.

The blood system is crucial for human survival. Every time the heart beats, blood is transported to all the vital systems of the body and its extremities. The purpose of blood is to deliver all the required nutrients and oxygen to all the organs and tissues of the body. Blood also helps with the removal of waste by-products. For the purpose of my discussion I will be referring to the blood and organs as the ***vital nutrient exchange system (VNES).***

The VNES is always on and its sole purpose is to deliver *vital nutrients* to the organs of the body. Vital nutrients are the key factors for human life. All the cells of the body require vital nutrients to survive and do their job. There are two divisions of vital nutrients: Macro and Micro. Macro vital nutrients are carbohydrates, proteins, fats, and water. Micro vital nutrients are sub-divisions of macro vital nutrients: including simple and complex sugars, amino acids, fatty acids, and vitamins, and minerals.

If you think of the Vital Nutrient Exchange System as a wheel moving in a constant clockwise motion it makes it easier to understand metabolism.

As the external nutrients are consumed via the mouth they travel down the esophagus ending up into the stomach. The stomach breaks down the food into smaller constituents. Digestive enzymes help break down food that enters the stomach. Once the finely churned food is mixed well enough, it enters into the small intestines as chyme for further breakdown and nutrient exchange. The intestines have two parts: large and small.

The large intestine is divided into six parts: cecum, ascending colon, transverse colon, descending colon, sigmoid colon, and rectum. The small intestine is divided into three sections: upper, jejunum, and ileum. The lining of the small intestine secretes a hormone called secretin, which stimulates the pancreas to produce digestive enzymes.

The material from the small intestine goes into the portal vein, one of two blood vessels connected to the liver. The other blood vessel is the hepatic artery, which brings oxygenated blood from the heart so the liver stays healthy and functioning. The liver is like a filter that establishes healthy levels for nutrients to pass into the blood stream. The liver is a complex organ that has thousands of enzymatic processes that produce amino acids, which are essential for body function. Cholesterol production, healthy and unhealthy, is developed by the liver. Overall, the liver's main job is to maintain equilibrium in the body.

Once the nutrients enter the bloodstream, they are available to feed all the cells of the body. Cells are made up of proteins that are living organisms, each having a certain function to perform. All cells in the body have the same basic make up; however, they differ slightly depending where they are in the body. The remarkable thing about human physiology is how all the cells form to make organs and tissue. Cells cluster to make up body tissue. Body tissue forms to make up the organs, bone, and muscle.

Each organ has a certain nutrient requirement that must be met every day in order for proper function and survival. The body is in a constant state of change. Every second of our life cells die and regenerate. Cell degeneration is a natural process and must happen. However, cell degeneration can be slowed down by establishing a rich environment of nutrients throughout the body.

The digestive process allows for external nutrients to enter in the bloodstream. The vital nutrients feed the vital organs of the body. Failure to provide vital nutrients to the body can result in illness or disease of the organs. It is important to provide proper amounts of vital nutrients every day to keep the systems of the body running efficiently. As long as there is a good external source of vital nutrients coming in via the intestines, then the body is able to remain in an ***anabolic metabolism.***

Anabolic metabolism is when the physiology of the body permits normal cellular regeneration and energy utilization. The cells are able to feed and grow. Muscle tissue is not used for protein synthesis. When the body is compromised and vital nutrients are not coming into the body from the intestines, ***catabolic metabolism*** develops.

Catabolic metabolism occurs when the VNES is running out of vital nutrients. The physiological systems, through a series of hormonal sequences, will shift the metabolism to break down muscle tissue to provide protein to the vital organs. Since there is an abundant number of muscle cells, the body can utilize these cells during times of malnutrition. The VNES is able to continue delivering vital nutrients throughout the body without disrupting the homeostatic processes. *Homeostasis* is the regulatory balance among all the systems of the body. The disadvantage of being in a catabolic state is that muscle tissue continues to shrink due to internal protein synthesis. *Internal protein synthesis* is the process where skeletal muscle (protein) is broken down to supply the vital nutrients to the vital organs. When muscle cells are used for protein synthesis, they lose their ability to metabolize fat. The result is loss in muscle tissue (atrophy) and gain in fat storage. Protein is crucial for the development of all the cells of the body. Protein synthesis is divided into two parts, macro and micro. Macro protein synthesis is the metabolism of food consumed broken down to feed the VNES. Micro protein synthesis is the breakdown of proteins into smaller units called amino acids and how they are used at the cellular level.

# Macro Protein Synthesis

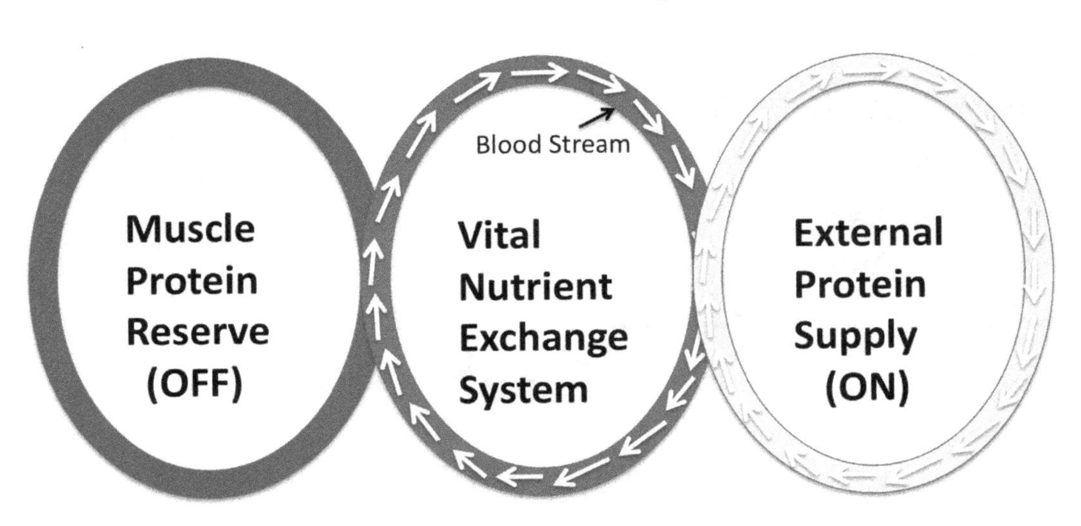


When external protein enters the body, it goes through the digestive system and enters the VNES to feed the vital organs and body tissue. There must be enough protein during the day to maintain anabolic metabolism.

When there is not enough external protein coming into the VNES, the body then turns on the muscle protein reserves to keep the supply of protein high enough to sustain the VNES. Catabolic metabolism is not a desirable state to be in for prolonged times. The result of catabolic metabolism is loss of muscle tissue and lack of fat metabolism. For example, if a person needs 150 grams of protein per day and they only take in 50 grams from external dietary means, they are in a deficit of 100 grams. A hundred grams of protein is still needed to supply the VNES. That protein will come from muscle protein. It is important to get the correct amount of external dietary protein to avoid chronic catabolism.

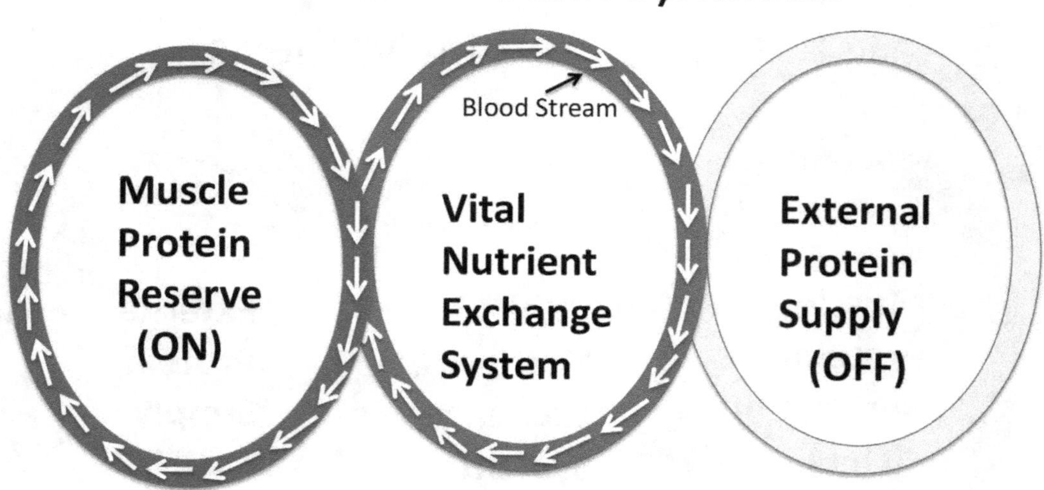


Once protein enters the body it goes through a cascade of events through the digestive system before it enters the VNES. It takes approximately two to three hours for the protein ingested to get into the VNES. When protein enters the bloodstream it remains there for approximately two to three hours. This is why it is crucial to maintain proper protein intake throughout the day to keep protein levels high in the VNES. Protein is constantly needed to repair and rebuild all the cells of the body. If there is not enough protein coming into the VNES via external sources, then the vital organs must depend on the skeletal muscle for protein.

Skeletal muscle tissue is necessary for fat metabolism. If skeletal muscle tissue enters catabolism, then fat metabolism ceases. During catabolism, the body goes into a defensive state. The defensive state is an innate survival mechanism that is in the human DNA that keeps the body functioning on a low level of nutrient exchange. During a catabolic event the body holds onto fat cells for potential fuel and vitamin exchange. The body can use large amounts of skeletal muscle tissue for survival if necessary. However, this is not desirable. It is important to keep the external protein supply on throughout the day to avoid using skeletal muscle protein reserves.

# The Process of Protein Regeneration

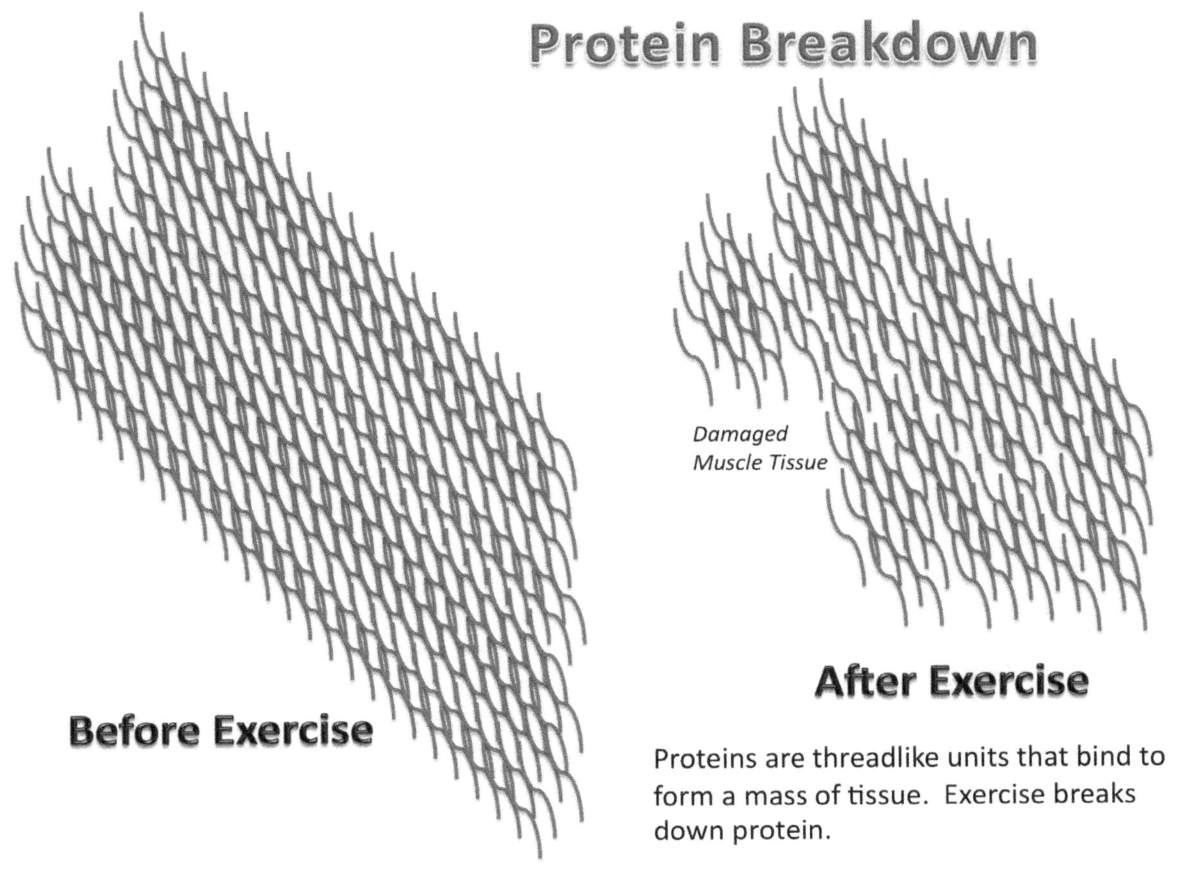


Exercise is a way to boost the metabolic processes of the body. During an exercise session the body tears down muscle protein. The more intense the exercise, the more muscle is broken down. This is a normal process. Once the exercise bout is over the body goes into repair mode. The protein must be re-established in order to prepare the muscles for the next exercise session. This is the concept of being fit. Being fit means that a person has greater adaptability to sustained increases of physical stress. A fit person can train the muscle hard and recover appropriately. The only way to maintain a good fitness level is through eating enough external dietary protein. The more you exercise, the more external dietary protein is required to repair the muscle.

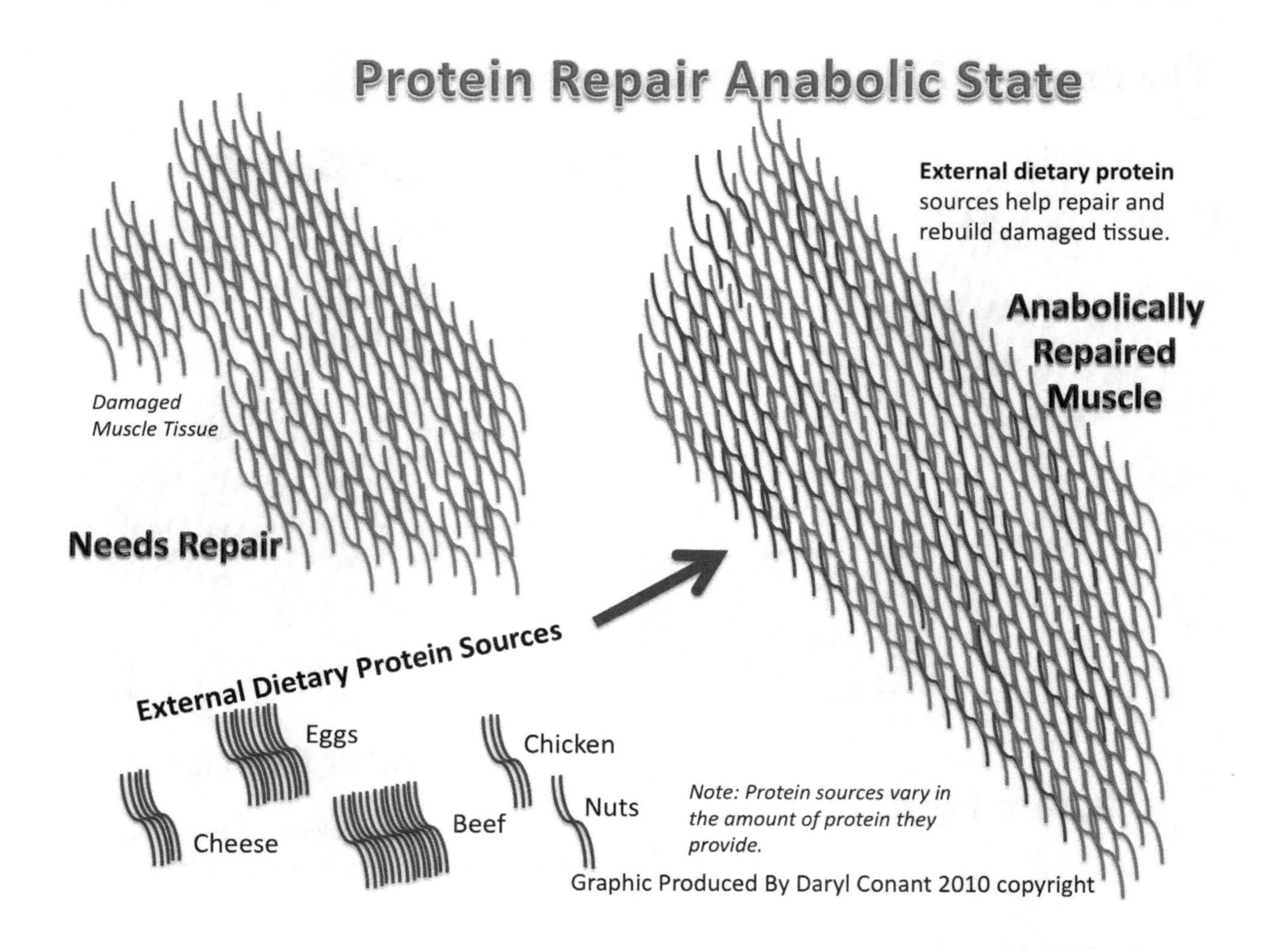


Consuming proper amounts of external dietary protein during the recovery phase re-establishes protein in the muscle. The greater the exercise intensity the more dietary protein is needed. When there is enough dietary protein coming in and the muscle is repaired, this is known as the anabolic state.

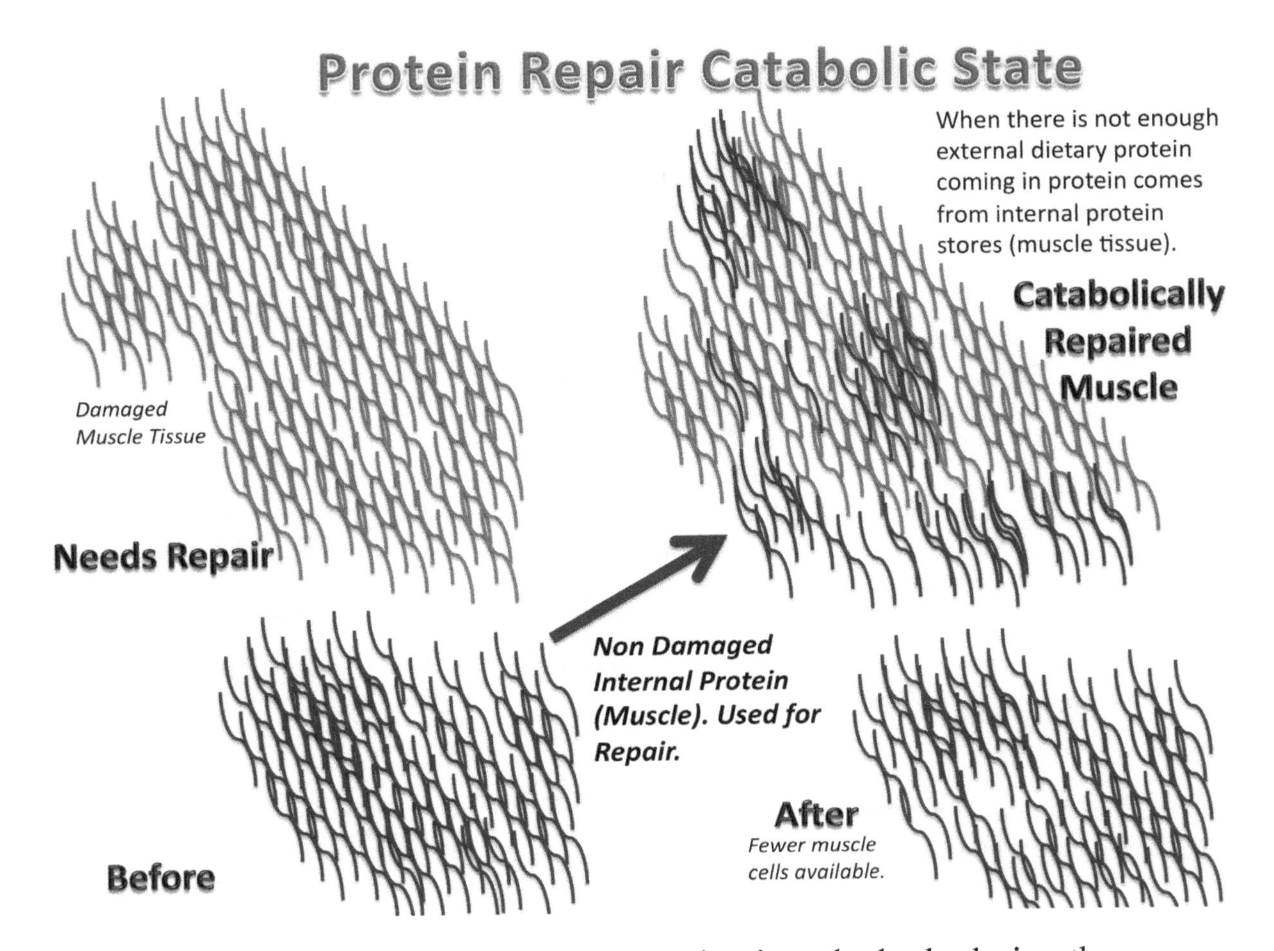


When there is not enough dietary protein coming into the body during the recovery phase, the body goes into a catabolic state. During the catabolic state the damaged muscle tissue needs to be repaired. Since there is not enough dietary protein coming into the system, the body must use its own internal muscle tissue to repair the damaged muscle tissue. This is counterproductive. Once the damaged tissue gets repaired, the non damaged muscle tissue has fewer protein units. It is important to avoid the catabolic state and to replenish the body with enough external dietary protein to keep the system in an anabolic state.

## Macro Sugar Synthesis

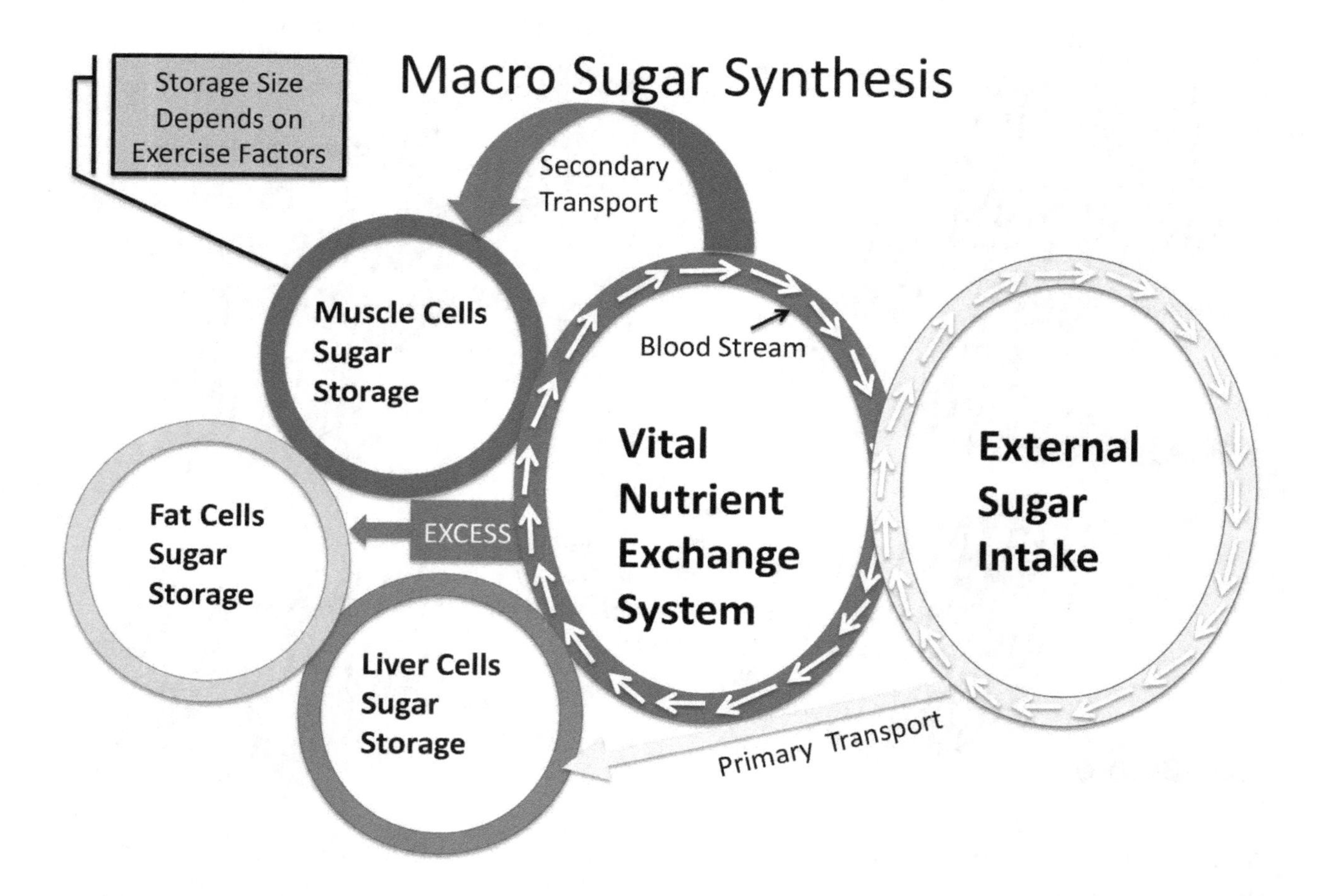


Sugar is an important part of cellular physiology. There must be an adequate amount of VNES blood sugar (glucose) to maintain homeostasis. If there is too much sugar in the blood it is cleared out by the release of insulin. Insulin activates cells to open for sugar to enter. When muscle and liver cells are depleted of sugar, due to metabolic respiration, they are restored by excess blood sugar. If skeletal muscle and liver cells have enough sugar, then excess blood sugar goes into fat cells. This is discussed further in the *Muscle Metabolism* section of this book.

***OBESITY IS DIRECTLY LINKED TO CONSUMING TOO MUCH SUGAR. Obesity is not a dietary fat issue, it is a sugar issue.***

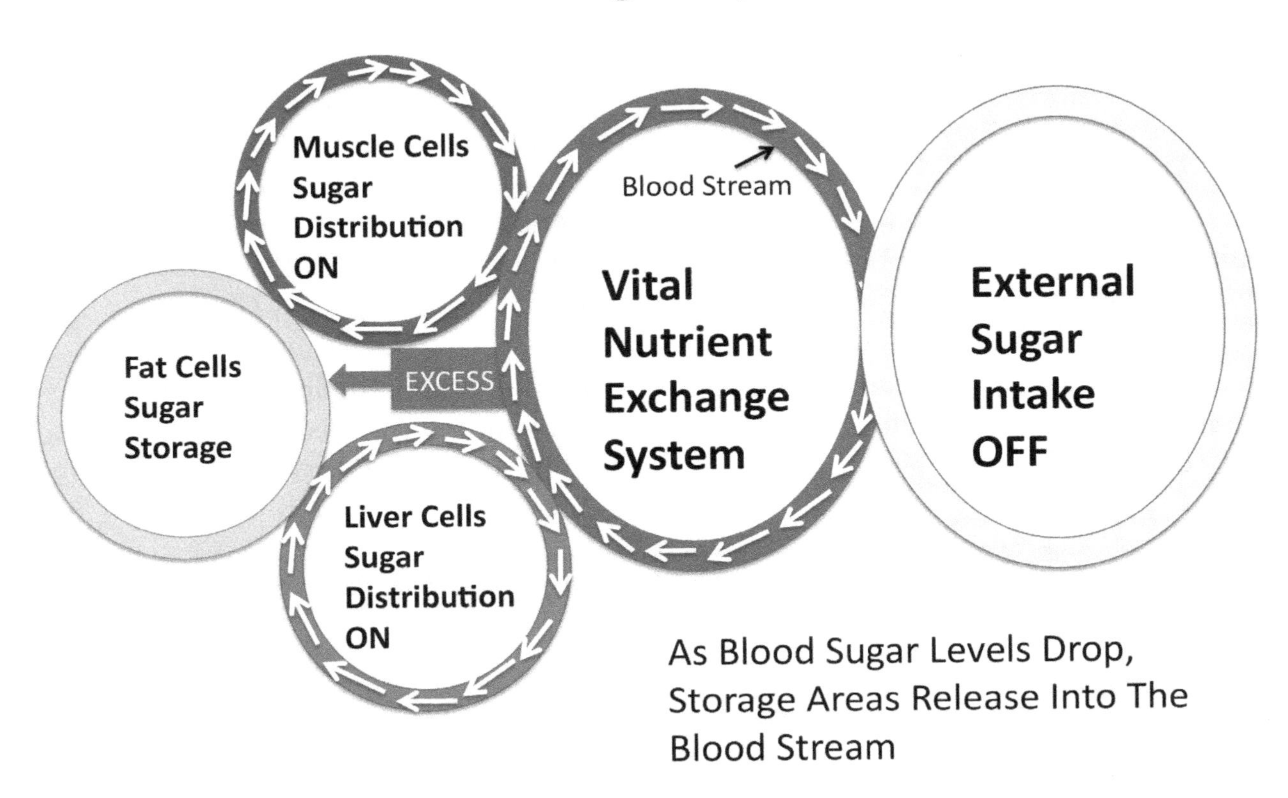


The amount of sugar needed to support the VNES is small. The amount of sugar that Americans consume on a daily basis exceeds the required levels of the VNES. Obesity is an epidemic in America that is increasing, and it is largely due to the fact that people are consuming too much sugar. When a person chronically abuses sugar, the VNES can be damaged, causing a shut down in the production of insulin via the pancreas. When the pancreas cannot produce insulin it is known as diabetes.

Diabetes is a serious disease that effects millions of Americans each year. There are two types of diabetes: type I and type II. Type I is known as juvenile diabetes because it affects young children and young adults. Type I diabetes is usually a hereditary condition. However, Type I diabetes can still develop later in life and is more prominent in white Americans than other ethnic groups. Type II diabetes develops later in life in both men and women. Age, lifestyle, and dietary factors can contribute to type II diabetes. Type II diabetics can still produce insulin from the pancreas; however, the cells of the body are resistant to insulin. Insulin is an anabolic hormone that clears excess sugar out of the bloodstream. Insulin forces cell receptors to open up to allow sugar to enter. In normal circumstances, the cells open and the sugar enters, stabilizing blood-sugar levels. In type II diabetes, the cell receptors do not open, because they are resistant to insulin causing sugar to remain in the bloodstream. High sugar levels continue to signal the pancreas to release insulin. High levels of insulin n the body is known as hyperinsulinemia. Hyperinsulinemia increases the risk of heart disease and other health risks. Those that have type I diabetes have to take daily insulin injections since they do not produce insulin from their pancreas. People that have either type I or type II diabetes can control their blood-sugar levels by maintaining a healthy intake of low glycemic foods and partaking in regular exercise.

When the external sugar source is not active and the VNES sugar levels get low, sugar from skeletal muscle and the liver is used to supply the VNES. Depleting the body completely of sugar is not safe and should be avoided. Glucose is the main

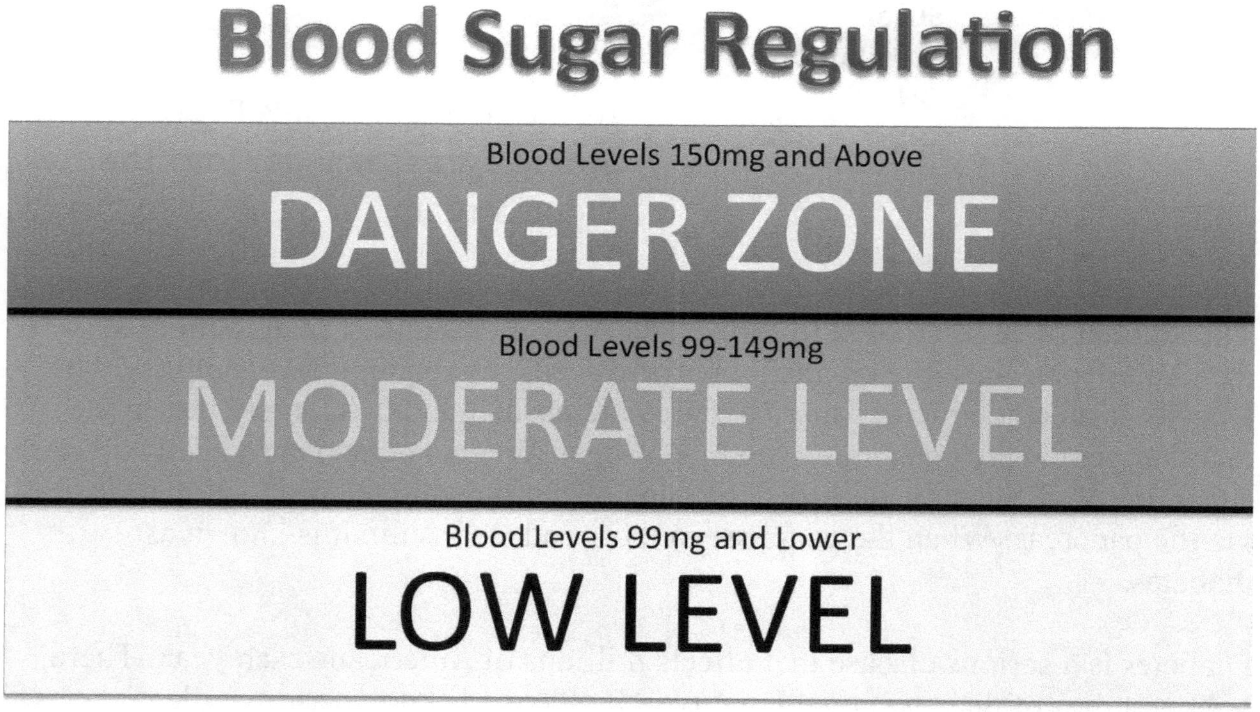

**Blood Sugar Regulation**

Blood Levels 150mg and Above

DANGER ZONE

Blood Levels 99-149mg

MODERATE LEVEL

Blood Levels 99mg and Lower

LOW LEVEL

Glucose is a simple sugar molecule used by all cells of the body for energy. It is the quickest acting fuel used in the body. The glycemic index is based on measuring simple and complex sugars to glucose.

energy source of the VNES and must be sustained in adequate amounts throughout the day. Though sugar is required for proper physiological functioning of the body, over-consumption can be damaging.

**Blood Sugar Regulation**
To help understand how much sugar the body can consume, it is important to know what amounts to dangerous, moderate, and low levels.

**The Danger Zone:**
Blood levels 150 mg and above are considered dangerous (hyperglycemia) and could result in illness or disease.

**Moderate Level:**
Blood levels 99-149 mg are considered the normal range of blood sugar. Maintaining 110-120 mg is optimal.

**Low Level:**
Blood levels 99mg and lower are considered too low (hypoglycemia). Blood levels too low are dangerous and could result in illness, disease, or death.

## The Glycemic Index

| | Example: | |
|---|---|---|
| HIGH GLYCEMIC | White Flour<br>Pototo without skin<br>White Sugar<br>Corn Syrup / Soda<br>Corn | Orange Juice<br>Fruit Juice<br>Cookies<br>Cake<br>Ice Cream |
| MODERATE GLYCEMIC | Carrots<br>Peas<br>Fruit with Skin<br>Sweet Potato<br>Milk | Yogurt<br>Sports Bars<br>Sports Drinks<br>Beets<br>Cucumbers |
| LOW GLYCEMIC | Whole Grains<br>Beans<br>Spinach<br>Broccolli<br>Asparagus | Greens<br>Meat<br>Eggs<br>Cheese<br>Nuts |

How fast a sugar is absorbed through the intestine and enters the blood stream determines their rating; high, moderate, low.

**The Glycemic Index**

The glycemic index ranks foods on how they affect our blood glucose levels. This index measures how much your blood glucose increases in the two or three hours after eating. How fast a sugar is absorbed through the intestine and enters the blood determines its rating.

Foods that are rated in the high glycemic zone are to be avoided. They produce ill effects in the body if overly consumed. The main staple of the American diet should be filled with mainly low to moderate glycemic foods.

**The Sugar Radar**

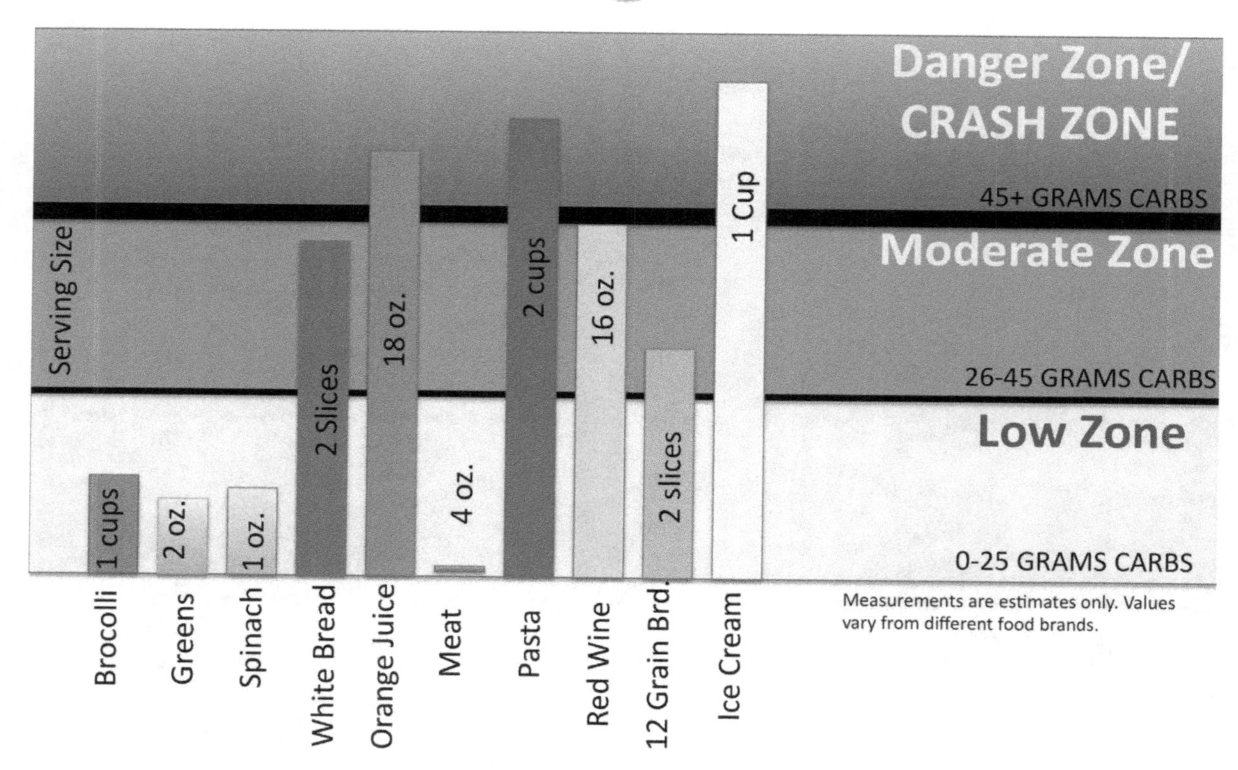


The sugar radar is something I developed to help you understand how much sugar can be consumed before it enters the danger/crash zone.

There are three levels to the sugar radar: Danger/Crash zone, Moderate zone, and Low zone.

Every food that you eat has a certain reaction in the blood system. All food has a glycemic rating. The foods that are rated in the high glycemic category (danger zone) get past the radar and cause a crash effect the fastest. The moderate zone are foods that should be consumed sparingly. Moderate zone foods pass under the radar. However, if over-consumed their sugar levels can get too high in the blood and set off the radar. Once the radar is alerted insulin is released. The low zone foods are the best choices. Low zone foods enter the blood stream very slowly and it would take a large quantity of these foods to bring the sugar levels up to the danger zone.

When you eat a food, you can avoid the danger zone by only having a smaller amount of it rather than over consuming it. You can eat just about anything you want as long as you don't set off the blood radar response. For example, ice cream is a high glycemic food. You can eat a tablespoon of ice cream without setting off the blood radar. The amount of sugar from one tablespoon of ice cream is not significant enough to alarm the islets of langerhans (pancreatic reaction). Broccoli

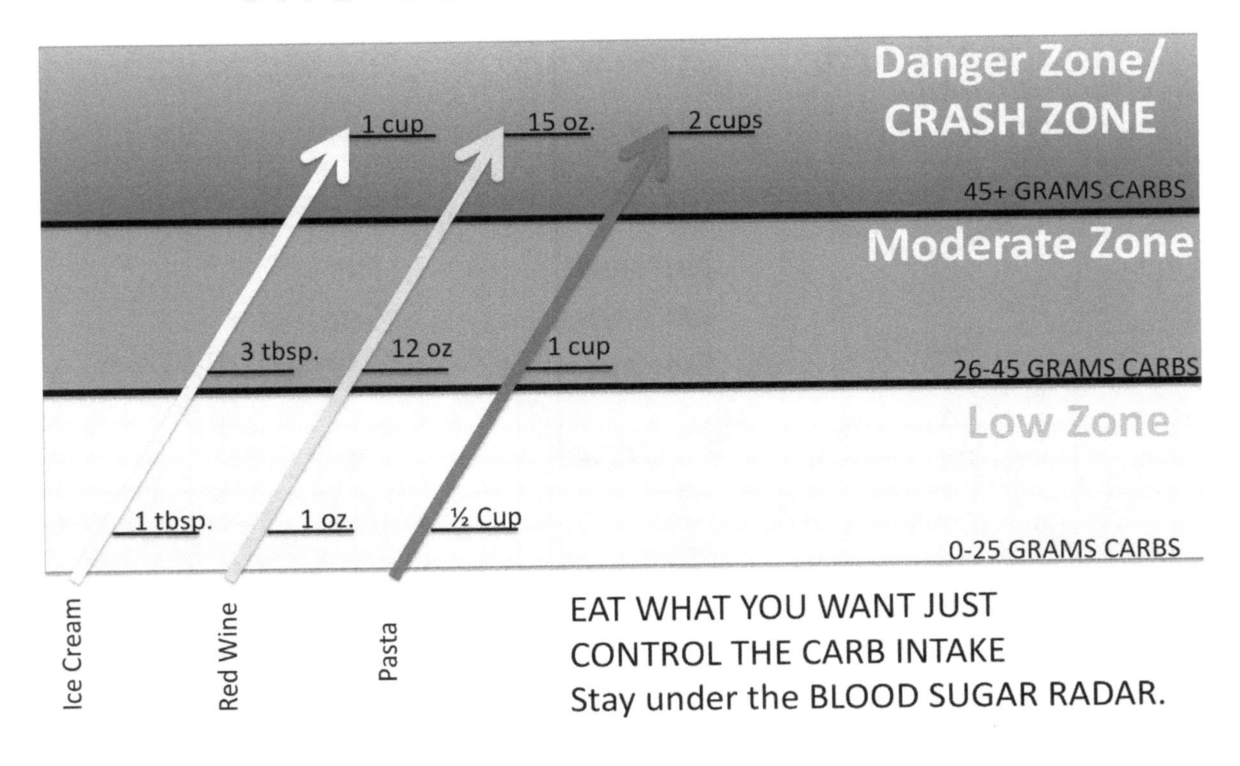


is alow glycemic food. You can eat two pounds of broccoli before it would raise blood sugar levels into the danger zone. Low glycemic foods are best because they must be consumed in large quantities to cause an insulin response.

**How Much Sugar Can a Body Store?**

The body can store approximately 300 grams of sugar distributed in skeletal muscle and the liver. During the day, we metabolize off a certain amount of blood sugar. Eating low glycemic foods throughout the day will restore blood sugar levels. The problem is that people are consuming much more sugar than they actually require. The excess sugar gets driven into fat cells. Also, high levels of sugar cause inflammatory conditions in the arteries and blood vessels. It is important to keep track of how many carbohydrates you consume in a day as well as knowing the glycemic index of each food.

**Fat Metabolism: Consumption of healthy dietary fat**

In order for fat to be released and burned, it must be activated by external dietary fat. When there is enough healthy external dietary fat coming into the digestive

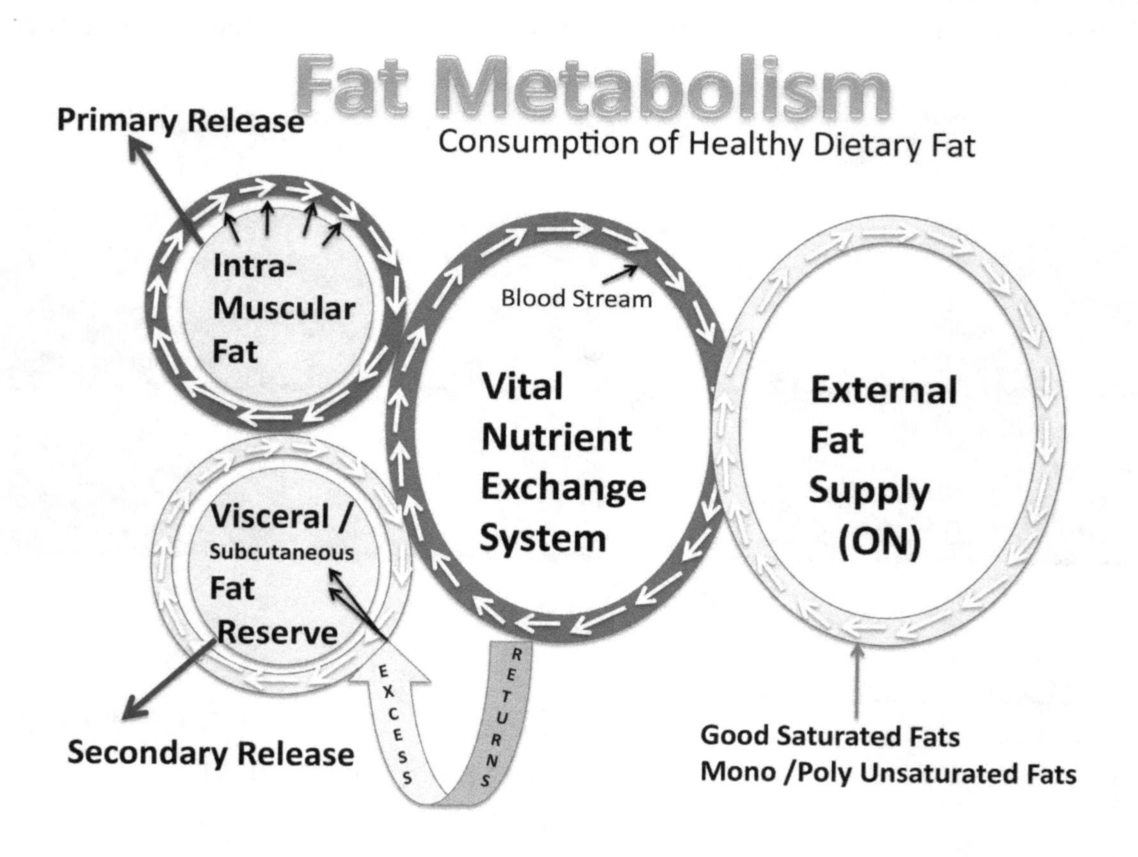


system, fat is released from the storage sites and metabolized. There are three different places where fat is stored in the body: intra-muscularly, viscerally, and subcutaneously. Intra-muscular fat usually gets burned off first, followed by visceral fat, and then subcutaneous fat. When an overly obese person comes in to workout they, get frustrated with not seeing results. What this person needs to understand is that when they engage in exercise the body is burning fat from the intra-muscular storage depots first. If a person has a lot of intra-muscular fat it will take them a longer time to see a change in the subcutaneous fat layers. The amount of intra-muscular fat differs from person to person. This could explain why some people see results faster than other people. They could have less intra-muscular fat and are able to burn from the visceral and subcutaneous levels more efficiently.

External fat is necessary to help the release of stored fat. The cells of the body have receptors that turn on and off when there is a certain amount of fat in the blood. If there is enough fat coming into the bloodstream the fat cells will release stored fat to be metabolized. The reason for this is that the body is designed to go into a deprivation mode if there is not enough healthy fat coming into the body. Fat will not be released from the fat depots when there is not enough external fat coming in. When external fat enters the bloodstream, it triggers internal stored fat to release and be metabolized in the muscle.

**Fat Metabolism: Consumption of No Dietary Fat**

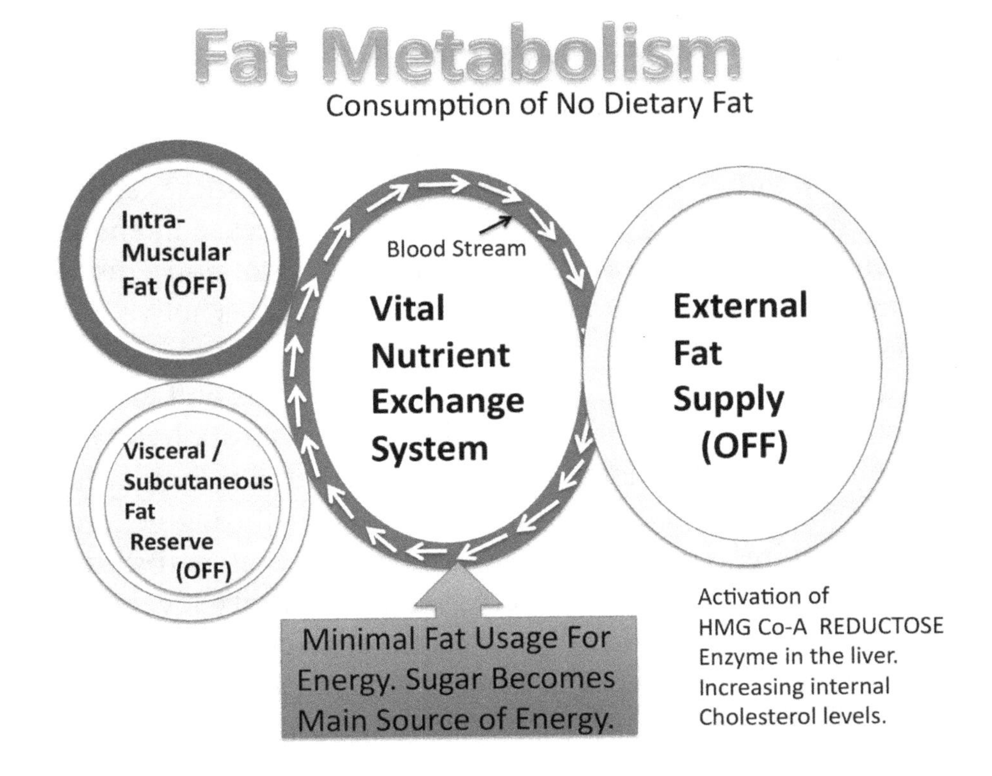


When external fat is not present sugar becomes the primary fuel source. Intra-muscular, visceral and subcutaneous fat reserves are turned off. The fat cells remain closed until there is a change in the blood fat levels.

# Metabolism: The Heat Factor

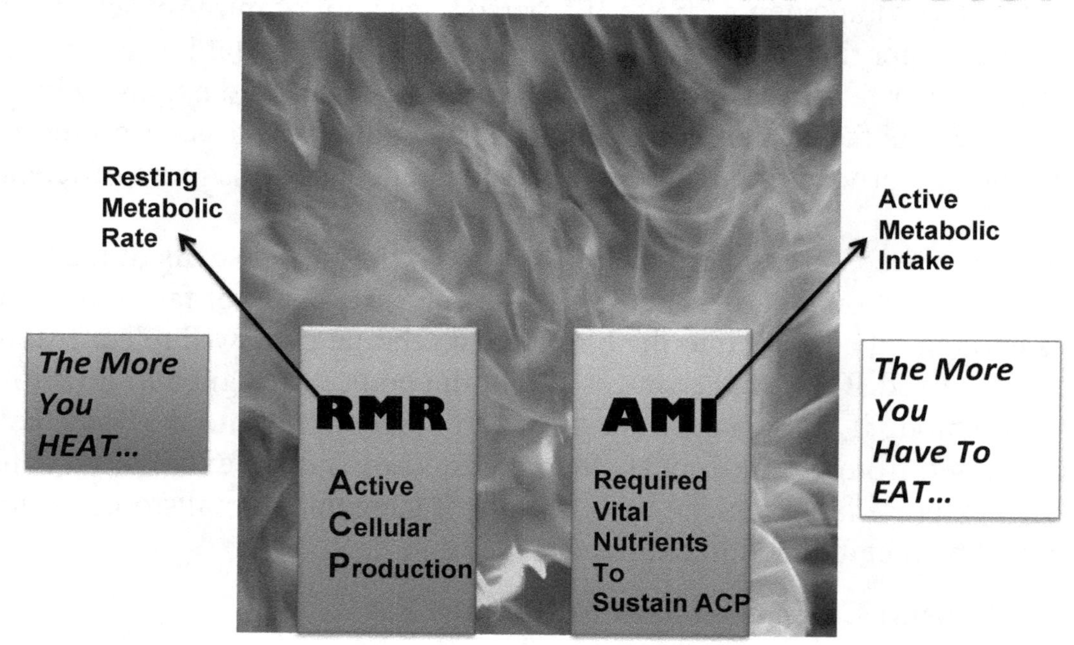


Now I would like to discuss metabolism. There seems to be a lot of different ideas when talking about metabolism. People think that their metabolism drops every year of their life. This is not true. I believe that VNES metabolism does not change throughout life. When we are young we are more active. We are running around doing more things with our body. Doing yard work, exercising and chasing kids around increases our energy production. This increase in energy production causes the metabolism to increase the production of vital nutrients. This is known as *active metabolism*. As a person gets older and is not as active as they once were, the metabolism demand is decreased. The body reverts to just maintaining the VNES. This inactivity causes atrophy of the muscle cells and thus decreases the fat-burning mechanism. When fat is not able to burn through the muscle tissue it is stored in the fat depots. It is not a metabolic issue but a muscular issue. When the muscle tissue is not being activated on a regular basis through exercise, the muscles do not require as many nutrients as they do when active and they do not metabolize off fat. Once the person increases their activity level (active metabolism), the muscle cells begin to burn fat efficiently again. To help you better understand how metabolism works I have developed a new concept of metabolism known as the Heat Factor.

In graduate school I was taught that to maintain body weight it was important to match caloric intake with caloric expenditure. For years I subscribed to this belief until I realized that calorie counting is ridiculous. Matching calorie expenditure with caloric intake does not work. Let's say that you are told to take in 1500 calories a day of food. You eat 1500 calories of sugar, thinking that you will not gain weight because you matched your daily caloric intake. Eating this much sugar, as we know, can cause many side effects to the energy system of the body and inhibit fat metabolism. Matching numbers for numbers is pointless. What we need to focus on is matching **A**ctive **M**etabolic **I**ntake (Vital Nutrients) with **R**esting **M**etabolic **R**ate (Active Cellular Production).

The ***resting metabolic rate*** is the amount of heat that is required for vital organs and skeletal muscle tissue to sustain cellular activity. The cells have a certain amount of energy requirement to function. The energy is produced by the cellular physiology of processing vital nutrients to repair, rebuild, and create energy. In order to satisfy the RMR there must be enough vital nutrients to match the energy requirement.

The ***active metabolic intake*** is the amount of vital nutrients required to sustain the Active Cellular Production (ACP). Vital nutrients are the main ingredients for sustaining cell life. Vital nutrients are vitamins, minerals, low glycemic carbohydrates, protein, essential fats, and water. Insufficient intake of these vital nutrients will compromise cellular processing.

The goal to maintaining a healthy body weight is to feed the active cells with rich vital nutrients. Every organ is like an engine that runs by itself; yet, they work together to keep the whole system alive. Each organ needs a specific number of nutrients to operate efficiently. The only way to supply the necessary amount of vital nutrients is from external food sources.

As long as the VNES is receiving appropriate amounts of vital nutrients and all the systems are working optimally, the resting metabolic rate remains stable. In order to increase the daily active metabolic rate, the body systems must increase their productivity. Physical activity boosts active metabolism. The amount of exercise and level of intensity will determine how long the metabolism will be elevated. This residual burning is known as the thermogenic effect.

## The Thermogenic Effect

The ***thermogenic effect*** is increasing the heat of the muscle cells to create a permeable state, allowing fat and nutrients to enter and be metabolized. The more muscle that is heated up, the greater the thermogenic effect. Think of it like this: Most of us have used a stove in our lifetime so this example will be easy to follow.

Here are the key components of the stove and what they represent.
Frying Pan = Muscle Tissue
Butter= Fat
Oven Burner = Exercise

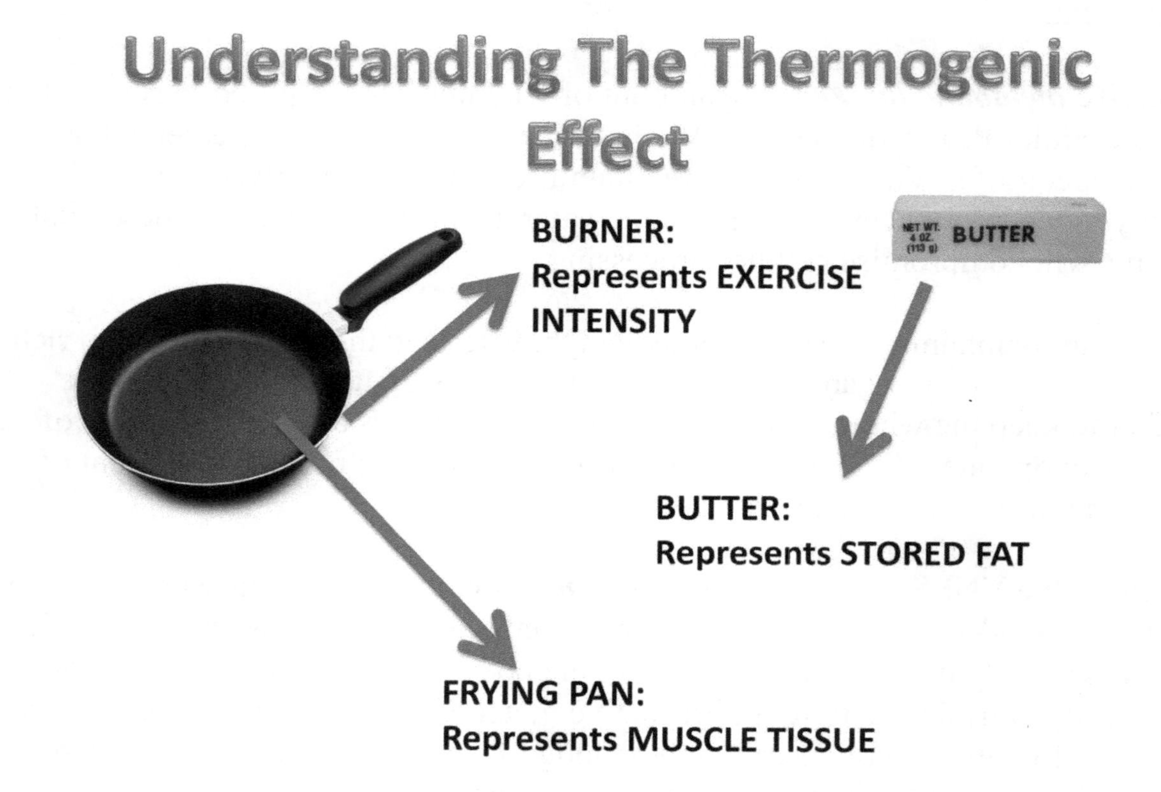


The goal is to burn butter (fat). First, you get a frying pan and put it on the stove. Second, you turn the heat on the burner. Third, you put the stick of butter on the frying pan. The butter will begin to melt onto the frying pan. Now, depending on how high up you turn the temperature of the burner will determine on how fast the butter will burn. If you put the burner on simmer (the lowest setting), it will take a little bit of time to melt the stick of butter. If you remove the pan from the stove, the frying pan will be warm but not so hot that you will get burned if you touch it. The butter will not get burned up because the heat is too low.

Now, if you place the frying pan back onto the stove and turn the temperature up to high, the butter will burn extremely fast. You will have to keep adding butter to the frying pan in order to keep the pan from burning up. The butter acts as a buffer to keep the pan from burning up and cracking. Once you remove the pan from the stove, the heat will be very high and you could get severely burned if you touch the pan. The butter still burns at a high rate in the pan even after the pan has been removed from the heat because the heat is so high. The continuation of burning the butter after the pan has been taken off the stove is known as the *residual period.*

The lower the heat on the frying pan, the less butter is burned, resulting in a shorter residual period. The greater the heat, the more butter is burned and the longer the residual period remains. The residual heat that continues after the pan is off the burner represents the **thermogenic effect.**

Understanding this simple frying pan analogy will help you gain a better understanding of the thermogenic effect. Exercise is important for boosting the active metabolism. However, the intensity of the exercise is important in determining how much fat is metabolized.

Here is how this analogy translates to burning fat in the body:

The muscles of the body represent frying pans. Each muscle group of the body acts as a separate frying pan. They can be individually activated to burn fat. Exercise helps to increase the heat of the muscles. If you exercise with low energy and low intensity (simmer), your muscles will be a little warm, but not warm enough to burn much fat. An example of this is when a person who gets on a treadmill and walks too slow, never getting their heart rate up enough to challenge the cardiovascular and muscular system. They stay close to their resting metabolic rate value. Once they get off the treadmill the muscle tissue cools quickly and the muscle permeability ceases. The thermogenic effect does not last long.

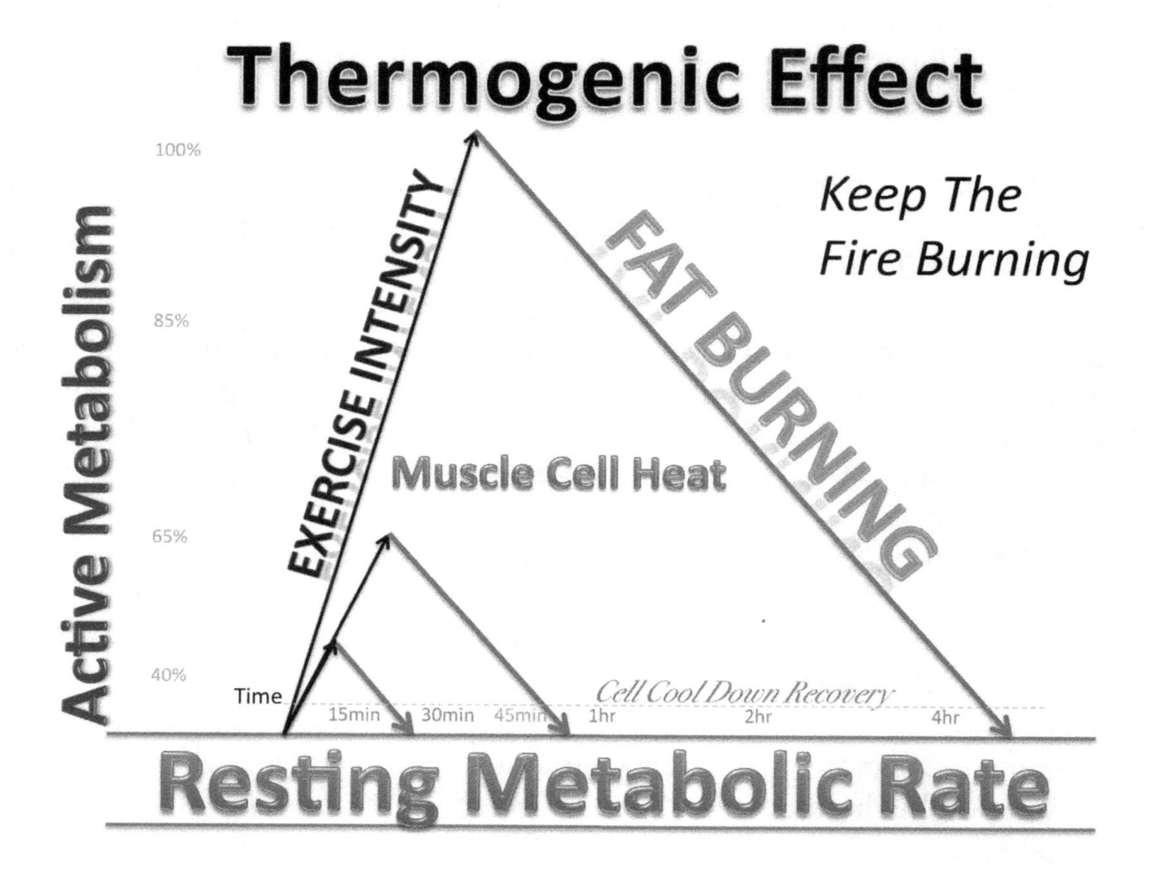


Now, if you exercise and increase the intensity (turning the heat up too high) the muscles will get very hot. You can feel the heat permeate through the skin when you train with great intensity. When you are finished working out (taking the pan off the stove) and driving home in your car, you still feel the heat of the muscles. What you are feeling is the thermogenic effect. Fat metabolism is increased during this period to help cool down the muscle. As long as the muscle remains hot, fat will be metabolized at a high rate.

The key to burning fat is to enhance the thermogenic effect by heating up the muscles (frying pans). The greater the intensity during the workout, the longer the fat burning process becomes.

The best way to increase more activation of the muscle cells is to exercise with enough intensity to tear down the tissue. It is during the rest and replenish stage that the damaged muscle tissue is rebuilt. Muscle cells will activate more cells to help with the load during greater levels of intensity. The more activity a muscle can produce, the greater the muscle is at burning fat.

Living a sedentary lifestyle will cause the muscle cells to atrophy (shrink). Atrophied muscle tissue metabolizes minimal amounts of fat; which is due to inactivity. To burn fat it is important to increase the muscle's activity to create more heat from within the muscle cell itself. Once you tear down the muscle it must be replenished with protein to grow and to maintain its high activity level. Active exercised muscle tissue craves protein. It is vital that you take in enough dietary protein after training to allow for proper repair of the muscle cells.

Exercising and not eating enough protein will only result in fat storage. This is because there is not enough dietary protein to replenish the torn down tissue. Catabolism of muscle tissue results, which is an undesirable effect. The best scenario is to exercise with the right amount of intensity and to replenish the

Activating More Muscle: ***The Anabolic Process***

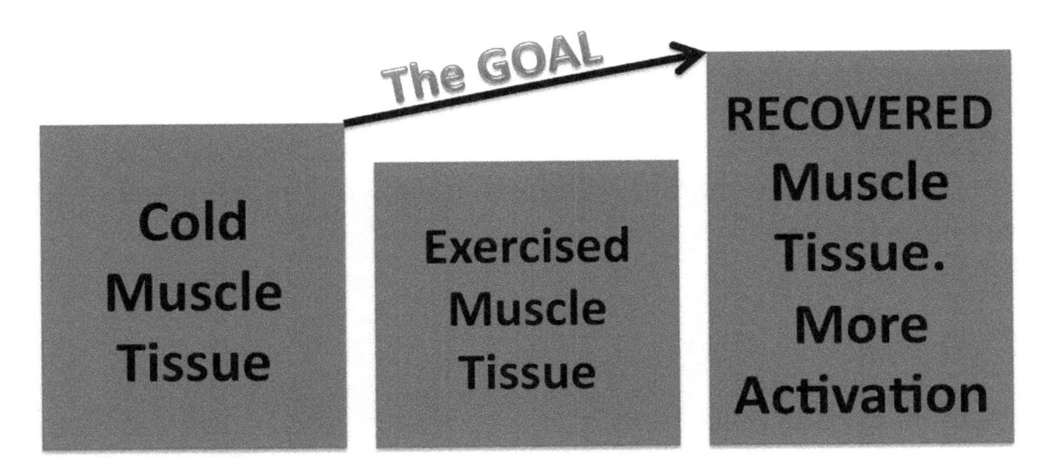


**The STEPS:**

1. **Tear Down Tissue**
2. **Rest / REPLENISH damaged PROTEIN**
3. **Recovered tissue allowing greater activation. Enzymes grow BIGGER.**

muscle with the right amount of dietary protein to allow for greater muscle activation.

# The More Muscle You Activate The More Fat You Can Burn

**Sedentary Lifestyle and Muscle Activation**

- Muscle's Atrophy = Fat Storage

**Exercise and Eat Little Protein**

- Muscle's Tear Down. NO rebuilding = Fat Storage

**Exercise and Eat The Correct Amount of Protein**

- Muscle's Tear Down, Replenish, Rebuild= GREATER FAT BURN

***Eat Like A Sedentary Person, Look Like a Sedentary Person...***

**Sample Exercise Programs**

In Appendix III you find more information on how to boost your active metabolism to increase the thermogenic effect.

# Factors Affecting Metabolism

Every now and then I get a client who just cannot seem to lose the extra body fat that has collected around their waist, arms and back. Even though they have followed the exact exercise, nutrition and recovery plan that I have prescribed, they still can't seem to change their body composition. If this happens then there could be factors that contribute to their inability to burn large amounts of fat.

The human body is perhaps the greatest system ever developed on Earth. Though we know a tremendous amount about how the body works, there is much we do not know. The systems of the body are so intricate and because they demand precise physiological synergy to function, if for any reason any of these systems are compromised, they won't work optimally which can cause imbalance within the body. Drug and alcohol abuse, hormones, food allergies, DNA factors, chronic over-consumption of food, sedentary lifestyle, ingesting too much sugar, and/or eating too little food can all be contributing factors of poor metabolic function.

If the systems of the body are compromised due the factors mentioned, then the chances of a person reversing their disposition is uncertain. Though not everyone is going to be able to burn off large amounts of fat and look twenty years younger, they can, however, help reduce the onset of producing more fat and inflammatory factors.

One time I had a client who was not able to achieve results with proper exercise and nutrition. I asked her to have her thyroid gland checked, to make sure it was functioning properly. It turned out that she had a very low level of thyroxine. Thyroxine is a hormone produced by the thyroid gland that helps increase the metabolic rate and regulates growth and development. Fortunately, she resorted to thyroid therapy with her homeopathic doctor. The damage was not as severe as in some cases. Sometimes the thyroid will shut down completely and cannot be saved. This woman was able to regenerate the function of her thyroid gland and start seeing results again.

If you are having trouble losing the body fat, I suggest that you examine all aspects of your body. I believe that everyone can burn fat. How much fat you can burn depends on the health of your body systems and hormone levels. There are many factors that can contribute to having a poor metabolism. Sedentary lifestyle, stressful living, lack of sleep, and drug abuse are some factors that can affect metabolism. However, there is one factor that is very seldom talked about and that is hunger hormones. Hunger hormones play a major role in the body's metabolism.

# Hunger Hormones and Fat Gain

You probably have never heard of hunger hormones. I am not surprised by this since hunger hormones have only been discovered in the the last several years. Hunger hormones could be the link between being lean and being obese.

Hunger hormones are activated during the feeding cycles of the digestive system. There is a strong link between the tongue, brain, stomach, and the intestines. When the VNES becomes low in nutrient, receptors of the intestines signal the stomach to turn on. The afferent nerves of the stomach send impulses toward the central nervous system. The signal travels up to the the hypothalamus. The hypothalamus is located in the brain just above the roof of the mouth. There is a section in the hypothalamus, known as the arcuate nucleus, that is responsible for regulating hunger, thirst, body temperature, fatigue, and circadian rhythms. The hypothalamus synthesizes and secretes neurohormones, known as hypothalamic-releasing hormones. The hypothalamic-releasing hormones activate or inhibit pituitary hormone secretions. This sequence of events helps to maintain normal eating habits to keep the human body alive. If there was no hormonal control and link with the central nervous system and digestive system, then the body would die. The connection between hunger and hormones is vital for life. There are two cell types of the arcuate nucleus responsible for controlling hunger and satiety. One cell is the Proopiomelanacortin (POMC), which activates the hunger response. The other cell is the Neuropeptide Y/Agouti Related Protein (NPY/AGRP), which activates satiety and helps increase the metabolic rate. The major hormones that are responsible for the activation of the hunger cells are PYY3-36, Ghrelin, Leptin, and MCH.

During the normal sequence of events, as the hypothalamus signals the release of hormones from the pituitary gland, the stomach releases ghrelin. Ghrelin does two things: first, it increases the desire to eat; second, it increases when not eating enough food. How the brain signals to turn off the release of ghrelin is by releasing leptin from the small intestines. During normal cycles, leptin signals the brain to stop eating. This cycle is normal and is how the physiological systems work in the body. If the eating cycle is disrupted by poor dietary habits or restricted nutrient supply, then damaging effects can develop. Once ghrelin and leptin are out of balance in the bloodstream, they cannot be reduced. These hormones will remain high in the bloodstream. This is possibly the reason why people who lose drastic amounts of weight by restricting their food intake into a dangerous level end up gaining all the weight back plus more. There is a strong link between gaining weight and hunger-hormone concentrations. In order to avoid the excessive amounts of hunger hormones in the bloodstream, it is important to cycle eating throughout the day. Eating five to six small meals will help maintain the ghrelin/ leptin sequence.

When the normal cycle of ghrelin is disrupted due to abnormal eating patterns and malnutrition, ghrelin increases in the blood stream. This can cause an insatiable desire to always eat. The same holds true for leptin. Leptin is produced by the fat cells of the body and it travels to the brain to help turn off the hunger cell. Leptin is responsible for satiety. The more fat cells a person has, the more leptin they produce. This becomes dangerous because high levels of leptin mixed with high levels of insulin turns off the cells that produce ghrelin. You might be thinking that repressing ghrelin is a good thing, because it would reduce hunger feelings. The problem occurs when the leptin levels remain high over a prolonged period of time. This causes the satiety cell to become non-reactive to leptin. The hunger cell thus becomes hypersensitive to ghrelin. The feeling one may develop in this situation is a feeling of fullness. People that skip breakfast are likely to be obese because they often don't feel hungry in the morning. This could be due to the fact that they have high concentrations of leptin in the blood.

Our genes have developed DNA coding that signals the brain to protect the cells from starvation. Hunger hormones play a major role in protecting the cells from dying. When forced to, the brain will figure out a way to shut down metabolism by releasing hormones. This is an innate response in all of us. Unfortunately, this sequence is being fired off for millions of people each year because of their self induced malnutrition. The brain interprets poor malnutrition as a threat to the cells and will release hormones to shut down cells. There is no difference among the people starving in a third world country or the obese people malnourished in America. They both suffer from the same hormonal sequence.

Hunger hormones play a major role in many aspects of health. Here are some of the effects on health in relation to hunger hormones.

***Asthma and Obesity***

When a person is obese they have high levels of leptin. This high concentration of leptin can lead to inflammation of the airways, resulting in asthma. High levels of leptin causes cells to be resistant to it. This can cause a decrease in the cell's production.

***Atrial Fibrillation, Colon Cancer, Coronary Artery Disease, Diabetes, Gallstones, Osteoarthritis***

Increased levels of leptin increases the production of monocytes in the blood. Monocytes are white blood cells that help with the body's immune system. Normal levels of monocytes are healthy, but if the monocytes' concentration becomes high in the blood this can cause an overactive immune system. An overactive immune system is more susceptible to losing its ability to defend against free radical invaders that lead to disease.

***Cortisol***

Cortisol is a corticosteroid that acts as a cell inhibitor. It helps increase blood pressure and increases the utilization of blood sugar. Cortisol is known as the "stress hormone." High cortisol levels can inhibit muscle and fat metabolism. The normal function of cortisol is to help activate the sympathetic nervous system awakening the brain. Cortisol is released during the early morning to help the body to wake up for the day. Once the person wakes up cortisol levels fall, allowing normal fat and sugar metabolism to resume.

Hormones are released by a cascade of events. The hypothalamus releases a hormone called corticotropin hormone (CRH). CRH activates the pituitary gland, which in turn activates adrenocorticotropin hormone (ACTH). ACTH activates the adrenal glands, releasing cortisol. This sequence of events is known as the HPA axis. A receptor (V3 receptor) located in the pituitary gland is responsible for regulating the amount of CRH in the pituitary.

Serotonin is important for healthy functioning of the brain. When serotonin levels drop it leads to depression and the V3 receptor is activated. When the V3 receptor is activated the release of cortisol occurs. Prolonged levels of cortisol result in high blood pressure thus increasing ghrelin, which, in turn, increases appetite and slows down the metabolic processes. Remember that when leptin levels are high in the blood the satiety cell becomes resistant to leptin. Ghrelin levels could be low but the hunger cells become hypersensitive. In normal circumstances, low levels of leptin turn off the HPA axis. But when leptin levels are high, the cells become resistant to it, thus keeping the HPA axis on constantly. This perpetual cycle will ultimately cause weight gain. Fat cells will continue to grow in number and size, and as long as this cycle continues the risk of obesity is high. Controlling the cycle and regaining control of brain chemicals will reduce and reverse the effects of obesity.

### *Dehydration*

We are always taught to drink water throughout the day. The importance of water is essential for maintaining proper blood levels, pH levels and cell metabolism. When water levels drop in the body, the body goes into a dehydrated state. In order for the body not to run out of water completely, the brain activates the V3 receptor via the HPA axis. When the HPA axis is activated, cortisol is released to help inhibit cellular metabolism and slow down metabolism which protect the VNES from losing its water supply. Not drinking enough water can influence the risk of obesity.

### *Immune System*

The immune system plays a major part in defending the body against free radicals, disease, and cell imbalances. Cytokines are chemicals that help clean out the blood of bad cells. When cytokines are high in the blood the immune system is overactive. An overactive immune system usually means that there is high level of free radical activity in the bloodstream.

Cytokines are made up of monocytes. Monocytes are developed in the bone marrow. Their main function is to attack foreign substances in the blood. Leptin binds to monocytes. Monocytes last three to five days and then they die off. Through a series of reactions, cytokines are released. The three cytokines that help boost the immune system are tumor necrosis factor-a (TNF-a), interleukin 6 (IL-6) and interleukin 12 (IL-12). When these cells are activated they help turn on and off the immune system. Due to the fact that monocytes die out after a few days, leptin doesn't become resistant to monocytes, they only stimulate them. This increases the levels of TNF-a, IL-6 and IL-12.

The problem occurs when leptin binds to fat cells. The immune system does not get turned off because of the release of adiponectin. Adiponectin is a protein hormone that helps regulate glucose metabolism and fatty acid catabolism. When the adiponectin level increases it binds to monocytes and decreases TNF-a, IL-6 and IL-12 function. Unfortunately, fat cells last a long time; therefore, the amount of adiponectin is low, which keeps the immune system overactive.

An over-activated immune system can influence the following:
Alzheimer's disease, strokes, asthma, allergies (food and nose/sinus), hypertension, hypertension, hypothyroidism, diabetes, fatty liver, cancer, increases acquired aging, arteriosclerosis, and osteoarthritis.

### *Insulin*

Insulin affects hunger hormones by decreasing ghrelin levels and increasing leptin levels. When ghrelin levels are low, appetite is suppressed. If a person goes long enough without eating, a starvation reaction results that will cause an in shift the levels of hunger hormones. During starvation, insulin production drops, ghrelin increases and leptin decreases, resulting in fat cell shrinkage. This may appear to be a benefit; however, once the person begins to eat again, the fat cells fill up again. In some cases fat cells double or triple in number and size once the person goes back eating large meals again. The body perceives starvation as a threat and will restore its fat cells to prepare against another bout of starvation.

Overall, hunger hormones control many facets of physiology within the body. The unfortunate problem with hunger hormones is that they cannot be reduced in the blood. Unlike other hormones that decrease secretive actions with age, hunger hormones do not reduce during the aging process. This could be the reason why the body develops high levels of fat as a person ages well into their 50's, 60's, 70's, 80's and beyond.

There are ways to control the increase of hunger hormones. You can regain control of the release of both leptin and ghrelin by eating small healthy meals frequently throughout the day, getting the required sleep, and controlling emotional distress levels.

# How We Digest Food

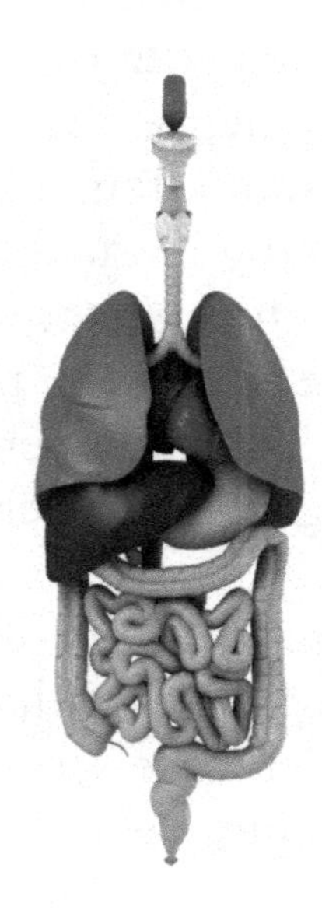

## *Healthy Colon and Digestive Tract*

The intestinal system is the major contributing factor for nutrient exchange. Nutrients must pass through the intestines to enter the body. Having a healthy functioning digestive system is essential for optimal health. If the intestines are polluted due to poor dietary habits then nutrient exchange is compromised, resulting in common digestive disorders such as: constipation, irritable bowel syndrome, leaky gut syndrome, and diaherrea. In addition, if the digestive system is compromised for chronically long periods, there is a greater chance for developing metabolic disorders such as heart disease, cardiovascular disease, and diabetes, which are all linked to manifestations of poorly balanced or poorly combined diets and years of digestive imbalances.

In our society, processed and chemically laden food, preservatives, hydrogenated fats, refined sugars, and exocitotoxins seem to be the staples of the American diet. By eating these types of damaging substances, the digestive system is subjected to poor nutrient exchange. By eating these chemicals, mucous material develops on the lining of the intestines and will reduce the nutrients entering into the bloodstream. The more you know about the biological simplicity of the human digestive tract, the more you can adjust your diet to ensure that minimum strain is put on your digestive tract and thereby reduce the risk for digestive ailments.

This will also help you to design a meal plan that will help the systems of your body rather than compromise them.

Why are there so many more digestive ailments today than ever before? The answer is simple--poor foods. I will try to explain this process as simply as possible. America was once a land where people harvested and grew natural foods: they drank non-homogenized milk, the meat and eggs did not have cement or antibiotics and steroids added, and the fruits and vegetables were free of pesticides. As the population grew, so did the demand for food. Farmers couldn't keep up with the demand of natural foods. Most of the foods, meat, eggs, and dairy that were produced only lasted for a short time, a week or less. This became a large problem for the country. The more populated the land became the faster our natural food resources were diminished. Then along came the idea of processing food and homogenizing/pasteurizing milk, adding steroids, antibiotics and cement into our meat, and using preservatives and other chemicals in food to make them have a longer shelf life. Now a gallon of homogenized milk can last up to one month on the shelf, where as non-homogenized milk lasted only one week. The bottom line in that the country had developed a way to spread out the food supply, but in doing so, also destroyed the natural make up of food. We all know that homogenized/ pasteurized milk is not the same as drinking non-homogenized milk. Homogenized/pasteurized milk is a poor food source and is difficult for the body to digest. Many people are allergic to homogenized/pasteurized milk. I can attest to this fact, as I developed stomach problems and allergies from drinking homogenized/pasteurized milk. Once I switched over to raw non-homogenized/ pasteurized milk, I never had any stomach issues or allergic reactions ever again.

There has been a lot of controversy about eating food such as eggs, red meat, and cream. It is believed that eating these foods on a regular basis will cause heart disease and high cholesterol. I have to disagree with this theory. I feel that there is nothing wrong with these foods except for when man tampers with them. Eggs that are not from a natural, free-range chicken are not good, because, in chicken coops, if the chicken is stuck in a box and forced to lay eggs, being fed man-made food filled with chemicals to increase the production of eggs abnormally, then the chicken is under tremendous stress, which raises the bird's cortisol levels. Cortisol is a stress hormone that protects the cells of the body by forming a barrier around them which helps stop the permeability of the cell. If cortisol is constantly present under stressful situations, then the permeability of the cell is compromised. Protein, fat, vitamins and minerals cannot get into the cell due to the stress response of cortisol. So if the chicken is under stress, the health of the egg is affected. Many of the proteins and fats in a non-organic non-free-range egg are poor, and in is some cases hard to digest in the human body.

Meats that have been injected with steroids, cement, and antibiotics are also poor in value. These tampered meats contribute to making people ill. Red meat is a superior source of protein if it is not tampered with. It is my belief that the drugs added to meat are what causes illness and high blood cholesterol levels. Many people, including nutritionists and doctors, are ignorant to the fact that natural foods do not cause illness; foods laden with chemicals, steroids, antibiotics, preservatives and exocitotoxins are to blame.

The first step to having a healthy, functioning digestive system is to eat natural organic foods. Get foods that are as close to their natural state as possible. The less the body has to break down the better the absorption of the food. A little common sense and knowledge of the digestive system and the food groups can ensure that you never tumble into the pitfalls of the modern diet. For example, it is wise to eliminate certain cooking oils that have been removed from their source, these include soy oil, liquid vegetable oil, or indeed any hydrogenated oil- simply because our digestive systems are unable to break down these oils into their constitutive elements.

Foods rich in such oils (mostly processed foods that need to use hydrogenated oil for longer shelf life) are said to form a film over the gastric lining, blocking the absorption of vital nutrients. This delays digestion and causes constipation. Oils eaten from whole sources such as nuts, are released slowly into the body, so no slicks occur. Non-hydrogenated oils also do not cause such adverse effects.

Alcohol also, can damage the entire length of the gastrointestinal tract and make existing ailments worse across the board. Alcohol has been implicated in the leaky gut syndrome and inflammable bowel disease and its effects on the mucosal lining of the stomach and intestines are known to exacerbate ulcers. Cirrhosis of the liver, for being so deadly and dramatic, consumes all the headlines, but the effect of alcohol on the digestive tract affects a lot more people. Directly or indirectly, alcohol affects the absorption of nutrients, interferes with metabolism and reduces appetite.

Your best bet to safeguard against developing digestive disorders is to eat healthy, natural foods and to stay away from antibiotics and non-steroidal anti-inflammatories. Antibiotics and non-steroidal anti-inflammatories are among the leading causes of digestive breakdown the world over. Antibiotics can destroy intestinal flora and allow yeast to overgrow, causing serious attacks of candidiasis (fungal disease). Over a period of time they can also reduce the body's immunity to certain bacterial organisms, greatly increasing the chances of contracting diarrheal infections. And for anyone with even the possibility of compromised intestinal health, a single dose of non-steroidal anti-inflammatory drug can increase intestinal permeability tremendously.

Other modern-day-style factors like stress and depression can wreak havoc with the digestive system. Juices are not secreted properly during such mental phases, not only resulting in excessive strain placed upon the glands secreting the enzymes, are that little or no nutrients are made available to the body. This is a dangerous scenario because you then run the real risk of being malnourished on a full stomach!

Remember, our bodies depend on the nutrients from our food not just for everyday energy, but also for repair and protection. Did you know that the GI tract already contains antibiotics that act as the first line of defense against infection? Or that it contains a major part of the chemical detoxification system of the body?

## *How We Digest Food*

**Step I**: Food enters the mouth. The mouth chews the food mixing it with the enzymes in your saliva. The enzymes help break down the food. The better you breakdown the food the better the digestive system will react. Chew your food until it turns into almost liquid form. Chewing food slowly will also help get the air out of the food, diminishing some of the ill effects of processing air in the stomach, like gas and bloating.

**Step II**: From the mouth food then passes down the esophagus. During the passage down the esophagus peristaltic movement occurs. This series of muscle contractions helps push the food down the esophagus. Through this contraction process the food is broken down further while heading into the stomach.

**Step III:** The food reaches the stomach and is broken down with the help of digestive enzymes. Hydrochloric acid helps to break down the three components of food (fats, carbohydrates and protein). There are enzymes that help break down proteins and starchy carbohydrates. Alkaline enzymes are used to break down starches and acidic enzymes help breakdown protein. If you eat both a protein and a starch together it makes the enzymes mix, inhibiting their effects on food. The food becomes a mix of both acid and alkaline which is hard for the body to digest. The intestines become compromised and it is likely the food will not be absorbed properly through the intestines. Therefore you will most likely eliminate the food without getting the nutrients you thought you were. This is why eating starches and proteins at the same time is not a good idea. These foods need to be eaten separately. The hydrochloric acid also acts like a disinfectant and prevents the overgrowth of organisms, both harmless and beneficial.

**Step IV**: After spending some time in the stomach-depending on what type of food you have eaten, the food turns into a milky substance called chyme. The valve between the stomach and intestines opens and food is pushed into the small intestine, broken into even smaller elements over a period of time.

This is where there exists a considerable interface between the blood and the gut by way of tiny capillaries. The broken-down elements and the vitamins and minerals all get transferred through the walls of the intestines, attached to carrier proteins.

Several other enzymes are secreted in the intestines. Secretions arrive from the pancreas and the liver. The pancreas secretes several substances that neutralize the acid secretions of the body. The liver secrets bile, which does not directly take part in digestion, but acts like a detergent; it enables digestive secretions to attack the emulsified fat.

In the entire twenty-foot tract of the small intestines, mucous is secreted. The mucous coats the walls to keep them from being irritated by the various powerful secretions. It also acts as a lubricant.

**Step V**: After all possible nutrients have been absorbed through the walls of the small intestine, a watery mix of undigested fiber is passed into the large intestine or the colon. The large intestine is shorter, about three feet in length. On average, about twenty ounces of digested matter enters the colon everyday. Of this, approximately sixteen ounces is water and the remaining four ounces is fecal matter. This is mixed up by the contractions of the colon and is stored in the form of a bolus.

Many digestive disorders occur in the intestines, especially the large intestines. These include ulcerative colitis, Crohn's disease, Irritable Bowel Syndrome and constipation. "Death begins in the colon" is a familiar phrase, but it is true that the colonic dysfunctions are suspected to play a major role in autoimmune or other degenerative diseases. Putting the colon in good working order is a high priority in the pursuit of good health.

# *Healthy Kidney, Liver and Gallbladder; Lymphatic System Function*

The kidneys regulate the body's fluid volume, mineral composition, and acidity. They do this by regulating excretion and reabsorption of water and inorganic electrolytes. This works to balance these substances throughout the body and keep their normal concentrations in the extracellular fluid. Ions regulated in this way include potassium, sodium, calcium, chloride, magnesium, sulfate, phosphate, and hydrogen. The kidneys regulate body fluid volumes, which are related to blood volume and the blood pressure in your arteries. The kidneys also regulate some organic nutrients and excrete metabolic waste products along with some foreign chemicals.

## *What does the kidney do?*
## *How does the kidney help regulate blood pressure?*

Regulating blood pressure is intimately linked to the kidneys' ability to excrete enough sodium chloride to maintain normal sodium balance, extracellular fluid volume, and blood volume. Kidney disease is the most common cause of secondary hypertension (high blood pressure). Even subtle disruptions in kidney function play a role in most, if not all, cases of high blood pressure and injury to the kidneys. This type of injury can eventually cause malignant hypertension, stroke, or even death. In normal people, when there's a higher intake of sodium chloride (salt), the body adjusts. It excretes more sodium without raising arterial pressure. However, many outside influences and kidney problems can lead to reduced capability to excrete sodium. If the kidneys are unable to excrete salt with normal or higher salt intake, chronic increases in extracellular fluid volume and blood volume result. This leads to high blood pressure. When higher levels of hormones and neurotransmitters that directly cause blood vessels to narrow are also present, even small increases in blood volume are compounded. This is due to the smaller area through which the blood is forced to flow. Although the increases in arterial pressure lead the kidneys to excrete more sodium which, in turn, restores the sodium balance, higher pressure in the arteries may continue to persist. This shows the important link between kidney disease and high blood pressure.

It is important to nourish the kidneys through healthy nutrition and supplements. Proper nutrition is of the utmost importance for healthy kidney operation. Soda, alcohol, refined sugar, high concentrations of hard minerals, and foods laden in preservatives and chemicals can cause a build up in the kidneys over time which could result in the development of kidney stones, kidney infections or disease. Since it is almost impossible to live today without being subjected to many of the harsh poisons that are in our food, water, and air, we must take care of our body systems in an effective manner to help the immune system fight off potential dangerous invaders. If you want to be healthy, you must have clean and healthy kidneys.

The kidneys, the body's natural filtration system, perform many vital functions, including removing metabolic waste products from the bloodstream, regulating the body's water balance, and maintaining the pH (acidity/alkalinity) of the body's fluids. Approximately one and a half quarts of blood per minute are circulated through the kidneys, where waste chemicals are filtered out and eliminated from the body (along with excess water) in the form of urine. Eating a diet rich in natural nutrients and staying away from as many poisons as possible will insure good kidney health. Refer to page 65 for a kidney cleanse schedule.

## *What does the liver do?*

The liver is a sophisticated organ that is the filter for the body. Everything that passes through the intestines must go through the liver. The liver breaks down the nutrients and decides whether or not they can enter the bloodstream. When substances are too potent to enter into the bloodstream, the liver will produce a series of enzymatic reactions to help breakdown the lethal substance to a less potent solution, that can then pass into the bloodstream. Poisons, like alcohol, are lethal substances that must be diffused by the liver before entering the bloodstream. If alcohol were to bypass the liver and go directly into the bloodstream it would be too lethal, resulting in a dangerous situation for the person. The liver diffuses the alcohol into a safer sugar compound, which then can enter the bloodstream. The more potent the alcohol solution is, the harder the liver has to work to defend against it. When too much alcohol is entering the liver, some of poison can't be stopped fast enough and enters the bloodstream anyway. This event will then affect the neurological systems of the body, causing a person to become inebriated. The liver is a great system, but can't stop everything that goes into the bloodstream.

If you eat poor nutritional foods and/or ingest large quantities of alcoholic beverages, the liver will not be able to defend against these toxic invaders. The function of the liver filtering system will weaken. Having a poor filtering system can result in a high toxicity of free radical invaders and poisons entering the bloodstream. These toxins can then harbor themselves in various systems of the body, which can make a person become ill. Depending on where the toxin ends up it could take months for the blood and lymphatic system to remove them from the body.

There is a direct link between poor cardiovascular output and a toxic liver. The cardiovascular system becomes compromised when the oxygen saturation in the blood is decreased. The liver is responsible for cleansing the blood. If the liver is clogged up with toxins, then blood flow is slowed down, resulting in less oxygen saturation for the bloodstream, resulting in poor cardiovascular output. Cleansing the liver of toxins can help improve the cardiovascular system.

A liver cleanse can help remove the build up of debris and toxins that affect normal liver function. Also, cleansing the liver can remove pollutants in the gallbladder and the liver and its bile ducts. By removing gallstones and liver stones from the body, digestion improves and therefore health improves. Clearing out toxins from the liver may also help eliminate common allergies.

One of the primary jobs of the liver is to make bile. It makes about one to one and a half quarts a day! The liver is full of tubes, biliary tubules, that deliver the bile to one large tube, called the common bile duct. The gall bladder is attached to one end of the common bile duct and acts as a storage reservoir for bile. Eating fat or protein triggers the gall bladder to squeeze itself empty of bile after about twenty minutes. The released bile finishes its journey down the common bile duct to the small intestine, where it helps emulsify fat. Eventually bile ends up going to the colon. Bile acts as a detergent to help digest protein and fats. Bile that is crystallized in the gall bladder produces gallstones, which inadvertently affect digestion. When an over-production of stones develops in the liver and gall bladder, less bile is produced. Gallstones can attach to bacteria, viruses and parasites that are passing through the liver. This is how an infection is formed; the body becomes infiltrated by newly formed bacteria and cannot be cured of these invaders until the gallstones are removed.

Performing a liver and gall bladder cleanse can help keep the liver and gall bladder working optimally, and possibly help safeguard against developing stones and other debris.

## *The Lymphatic System Cleanse*

The lymphatic system is where all the toxins from the body enter and are eventually removed from the body. Lymph is a thick, slow moving substance that helps clean the blood system. We have thousands of lymph nodes in our body that collect and help fight viruses and bacteria that invade the body.

There are three primary functions to the lymphatic system. First, it returns excess interstitial fluid to the blood. Of the fluid that leaves the capillaries, about ninety percent is returned. The ten percent that does not return becomes part of the interstitial fluid that surrounds the tissue cells. Small protein molecules may leak through the capillary wall, increasing the osmotic pressure of the interstitial fluid. This inhibits the return of fluid into the capillaries and tends to accumulate fluid in the tissue spaces. If this continues, blood volume and blood pressure decrease significantly and the volume of tissue fluid increases, which results in edema (swelling). Lymph capillaries pick up the excess interstitial fluid and proteins and return them to the venous blood. After the fluid enters the lymph capillaries, it is called lymph.

The second function of the lymphatic system is the absorption of fats and fat-soluble vitamins from the digestive system and the transport of these substances to the venous circulatory system. The intestines are lined with a material known as mucosa. The mucosa is lined with villi, small finger-like projections. There are two distinct types of capillaries in the lymphatic system: lymph capillaries, known as laceals, and blood capillaries. Both of these are found in the center of each villus. The job of the blood capillaries is to absorb all nutrients, except for fats and fat soluble vitamins. These two nutrients are absorbed by the lacteals. The lymph that is in the lacteals is called chyle. Chyle is a milky substance that has a high fat content.

The third and major function of the lymphatic system is to defend against free radical invaders, pollutants, and disease. A lymphatic cleanse can help remove and prevent the toxic invaders from taking over. It is important to know that a compromised immune system can result in the onset of disease. Taking the right steps to cleanse the lymphatic system can help boost the immune system and provide better overall functioning of the body.

## *A Healthy Heart and Lung System*

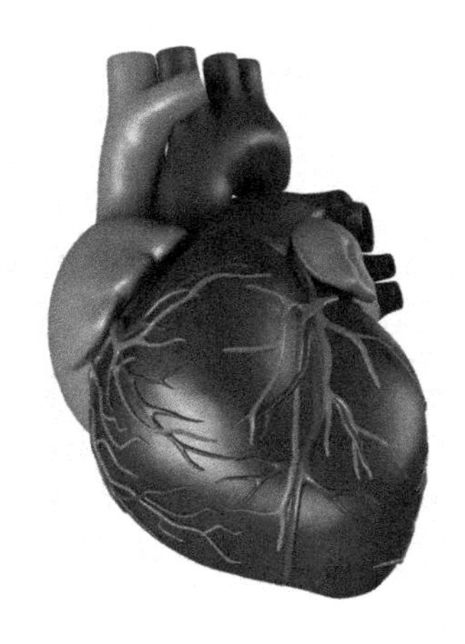

**Heart**

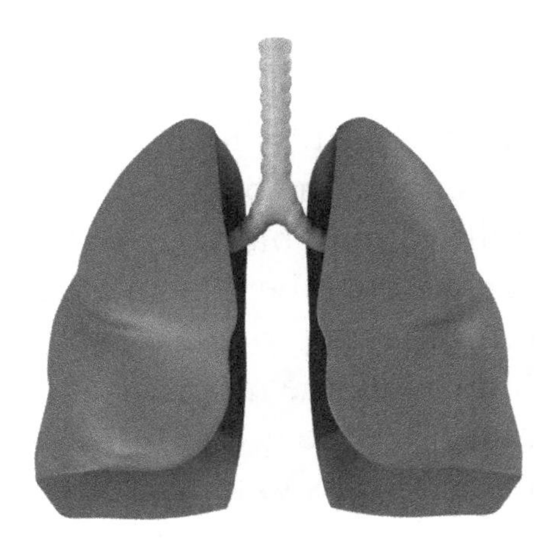

**Lungs**

Everyone knows what the heart does. The heart is an electrical pump that circulates blood throughout the body. The origin of the heart is a mystery. However, the heart contains the power to keep the body alive. The heart deserves respect and is often taken for granted. I am amazed at how ignorant people are when it comes to their own heart. They have no idea what the heart is made of or where the heart is located. Most people point to the upper right chest region when asked where the heart is, when in fact the heart lies more medial and under the sternum. People take their life for granted and are unaware of the magnificent power of the heart. People who eat poorly and ingest poisons on a regular basis increase the risk of developing disease. A poor diet and inactive lifestyle can influence the onset of plaque build up in the arteries. Once the arteries become occluded, the heart begins to starve, resulting in oxygen deprivation known as a heart attack. To avoid an early exit, one should adhere to a nutrient rich diet, exercise, and have control of their emotional state. Chronic emotional stress can be a contributor to heart disease. Taking drugs (steroids) can influence heart disease as well. Take care of your heart or else you will no longer be around to train another day.

The lungs work hand in hand with the heart. The lungs bring in the oxygen from outside and delivers it to the bloodstream, which then goes to the heart to be pumped throughout the body. Having a good lung capacity will allow for more oxygen to enter into the body. Remember, oxygen burns fat. The greater your lung and heart system functions, the more oxygen can get to the muscles to burn fat. To keep the lungs healthy, avoid first and second hand smoking, environmental pollutants and inhaling chemicals and chlorine.

To be successful in a healthy eating program, it is crucial to keep the internal organs functioning optimally. Cleansing the vital systems will ensure that all the systems of the body work more efficiently and synergistically. Muscle cannot be built without blood, and if the blood system is filled with toxins, poor fats, refined sugars, etc., then the muscle will not grow. A blood system rich in nutrients and oxygen will provide a great pump to both the muscle and cardiovascular system. Improving the recovery and repair of worked muscle tissue will ultimately help muscle tissue grow in size. In order to have nutrient dense and oxygenated blood, the gateways to the blood must work efficiently. The digestive system, liver, kidneys, and lymphatic system are vital to the production of healthy blood and body functions. Cleansing these systems throughout the year can dramatically boost the immune system and blood system and help support greater muscle gains.

## *Healthy Brain*

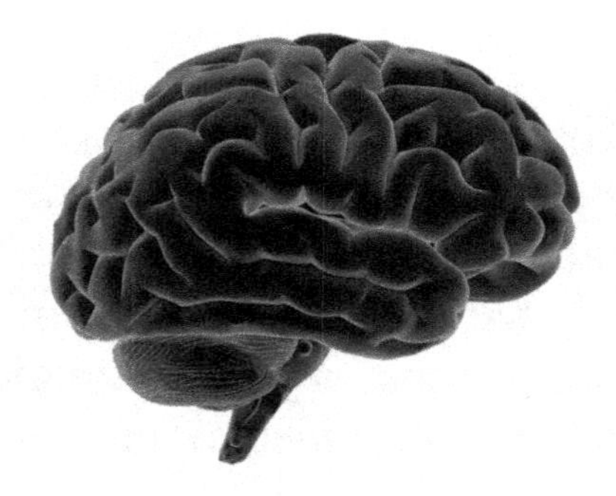

The brain is the control center of the body. It is essential to have the right amount of nutrients in the body at all times to keep the brain working optimally. Healthy fats nourish the brain cells and keep the neurons working effectively to communicate with the muscles to provide the best contractions possible. Ingestion of poisons from poor diets will contribute to damage of the brain cells and will result in poor production of muscle and other systems. If all the systems are healthy and working synergistically, in balance, then the brain will reap the rewards. Oxygen passed through the lung and respiratory system will be delivered to the brain to keep it healthy. The brain is a muscle and must be worked like any other muscle to operate effectively. If the brain is neglected, then disease and disorders can develop.

## *Healthy Teeth*

Keeping the teeth clean and free of plaque is important. Plaque accumulated on the teeth can pose a threat to the cardiovascular system. Plaque can break off and enter the blood stream via the gums. Over time plaque can contribute to the clogging of the arteries (arteriosclerosis) which can result in a heart attack. Healthy gums and teeth free of plaque can help fight against heart disease. Another reason to keep the teeth clean is to reduce the bacteria that forms in the mouth from eating food. Gingivitis and halitosis are two common problems that occur when the teeth are not clean. Gingivitis is the disease of the gums. Teeth can actually rot out of the mouth. Halitosis, causing bad breath, develops from a build up of bacteria either in the mouth or the intestines. There is nothing more distracting to a good looking physique than when a person opens their mouth and are missing teeth or have brown colored teeth. Keep the teeth healthy and clean for a better personal presentation. Avoid too much fluoride. Fluoride has been linked to breaking down calcium in the body. Toothpaste containing hydrogen-peroxide is more preferable for brushing teeth. You can even use baking soda.

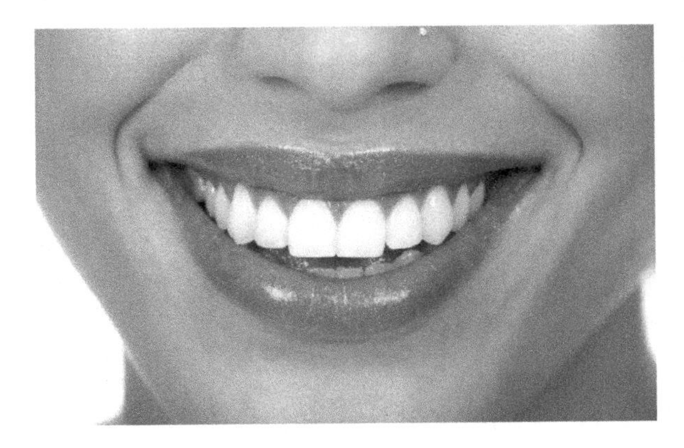

**Here is the Detoxifying and Cleansing Program. Developed by Ron Kosloff.**

**Step 1 Colon**
1st Step
5 Day Colon Cleansing Kit
(Complete full 5 Days)
2nd Step
Take 6 Lacto-zyme tabs per day for 30 days (2B-2L-2D) after colon kit is finished.

**Step 2 & 3 Liver and Gallbladder**
1st Week
Livotrit Plus (2B-2L-2D)
Beta-TCP (1B-1L-1D)
2nd Week
Livotrit Plus (4B-4L-4D)
Beta-TCP (3B-3L-3D)
3rd Week
Livotrit Plus (6B-6L-6D)
Beta-TCP (3B-3L-3D)

**Ultra P.P.1 -1** Dropper full per day

**Step 4 Kidneys**
Drink only distilled water for 10 to 12 days

**Renal Plus**
1st Week (1B-1L-1D)
2nd Week (2B-2L-2D)
3rd Week (2B-2L-2D)

**Argizyme**
1st Week (1B-1L-1D)
2nd Week (2B-2L-2D)
3rd Week (2B-2L-2D)

**Step 5 Lymph Nodes**
Choline and Inositol
(Fat Burner)

**1st Week**
(1B-1L-1D-1 Snack)
**2nd Week**

(Same)
**3rd Week**
(Same)
**Lymphatic Drainage**
2 Capful's per day until finished (1B-1D)
**IAG**
1 teaspoon (B-L-D)
**Thymex**
(2B-2L-2D) for 3 weeks

**Step 6 for 6 Weeks**
**Artery Cleansing**
**Porphyra-zyme**
6 weeks (4B-4L-4D)
**Cyruta-Plus**
6 Weeks (2B-2L-2D)
**Niacinamide**
6 Weeks (1B-1D)

Symbol:
**B= Breakfast**
**L= Lunch**
**D= Dinner**

**Caution:** If you return to your old eating habits of white sugar-flour-rice, hydrogenated fats, processed and refined flours, fried foods, fast food, soda, etc., then your efforts in doing these cleanses will be futile and your toxicity and congestion of organs will just return. Let this be the first step or the next step in total wellness for you! I know you will be pleased with the way you feel after completing this program. Thanks, Ron Kosloff, Owner NSP Products:

To order these supplements and supplements mentioned earlier in the previous chapters, call: 1(313)372-1807. Tell him I referred you.

Ron Kosloff is one of the most honest and sincere people I have ever known. I owe him a great deal for the wealth of knowledge he has given me. He sparked my desire to search for the truth about exercise and nutrition. Ron is one of my biggest influences in my career. Thank you, Ron.
**Please note:** *Consult your doctor before performing a cleanse of any kind. Be safe! Learn as much as possible about cleansing before starting.*

# Muscle Metabolism: The Mechanism For Fat Burning

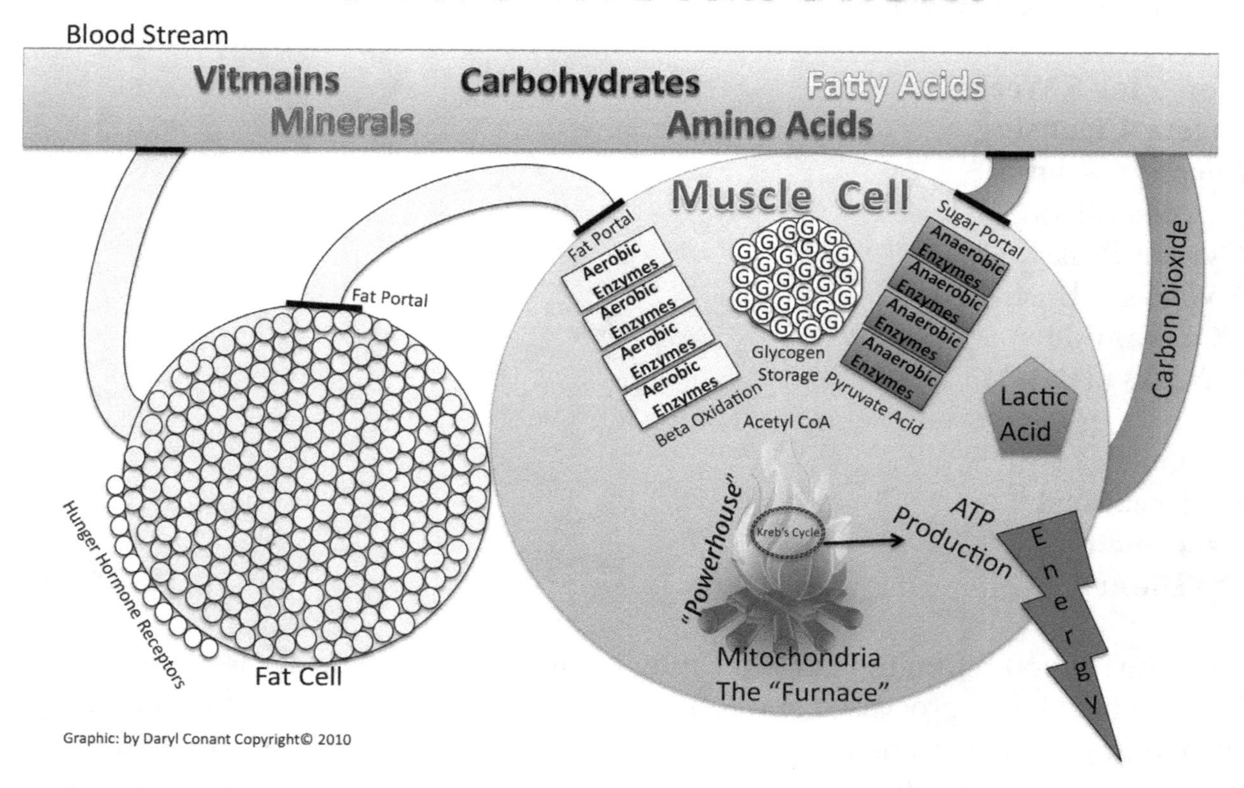


Graphic: by Daryl Conant Copyright© 2010

In order to fully understand how to lose body fat, it is important to know how the muscle works in metabolizing fat and carbohydrates.

The composition of a muscle cell is divided into two parts: organelles and enzymes (proteins). Organelles are tiny structures within the cell that have a specific function. Without getting too technical: I will discuss one organelle that is very important in the process of burning fat: the mitochondrion.

The mitochondrion is considered the "power organelle" because it is where the high phosphate adenosine triphosphate (ATP) compound is manufactured. Muscle metabolism is crucial for developing ATP. ATP is the main source of energy in the body and without ATP you cannot live. Fat and sugar help the production of ATP in a muscle cell.

Muscle metabolism is the key to burning fat in the body. If muscle cells are dormant and inactive, then the amount of fat that is burned is decreased. To burn fat, it must be metabolized through the muscle cell. The muscle cell has two types of metabolic enzymes: anaerobic and aerobic. Both of these enzymes can decrease and increase in size depending on the activity of the muscle. An inactive muscle (sedentary) or atrophied muscle will have small anaerobic and aerobic enzymes, low ATP output, low myoglobin concentration, greater sensitivity to lactic acid

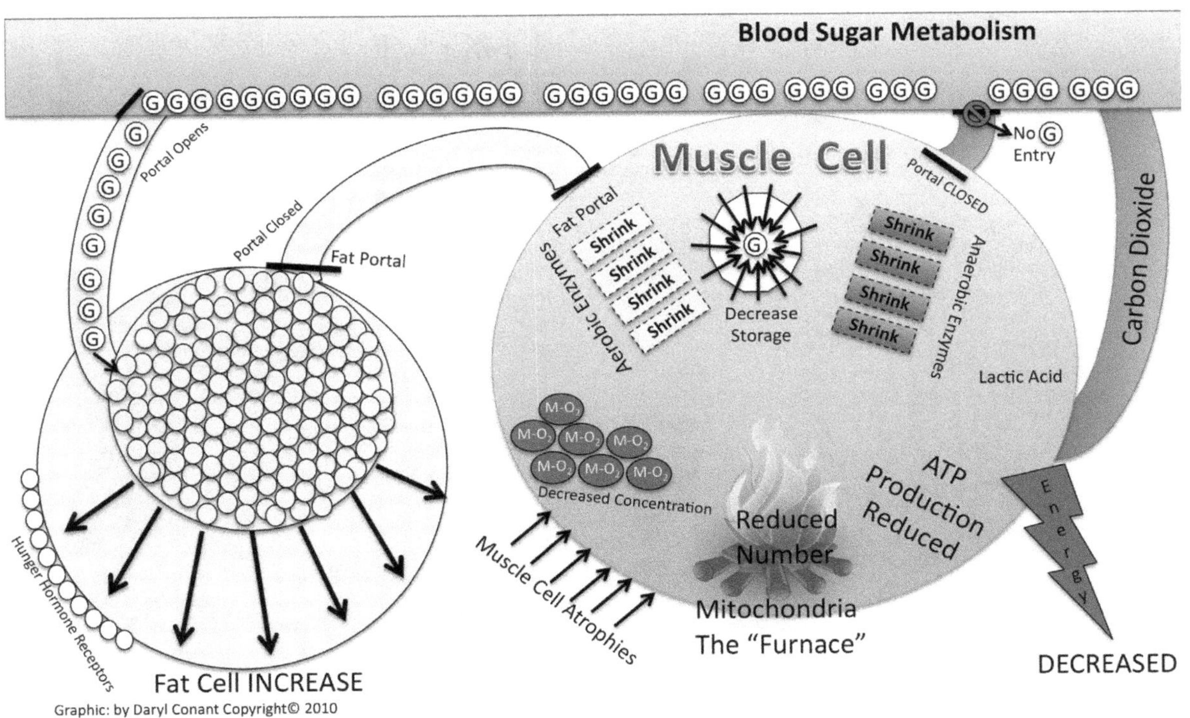


build up, and decreased glycogen (sugar) storage. Another disadvantage of having inactive muscle cells is decreased blood-sugar uptake, which is when blood glucose becomes too high and needs to be cleared out; insulin will be released causing increased cellular permeability. In conditioned muscle cells the insulin receptors open up the portals of the cell to allow sugar to enter into the cell to be either burned or stored. However, if the muscle cell is inactive, the glucose won't be able to enter the muscle cell and will be diverted to the nearest fat cell. A fat cell can store both fat molecules and glucose molecules. Once the glucose molecule enters a fat cell, it turns into fat.

An active and conditioned muscle will have greater ATP production, greater myoglobin (muscle oxygen) concentration, bigger and increased number of mitochondria, increased lactate threshold, increased glycogen storage, increased size of other organelles, and bigger anaerobic and aerobic enzymes. The bigger the enzymes, the more fat and sugar can be used in the cell, providing for greater ATP output. The more ATP you have the more energy you can produce.

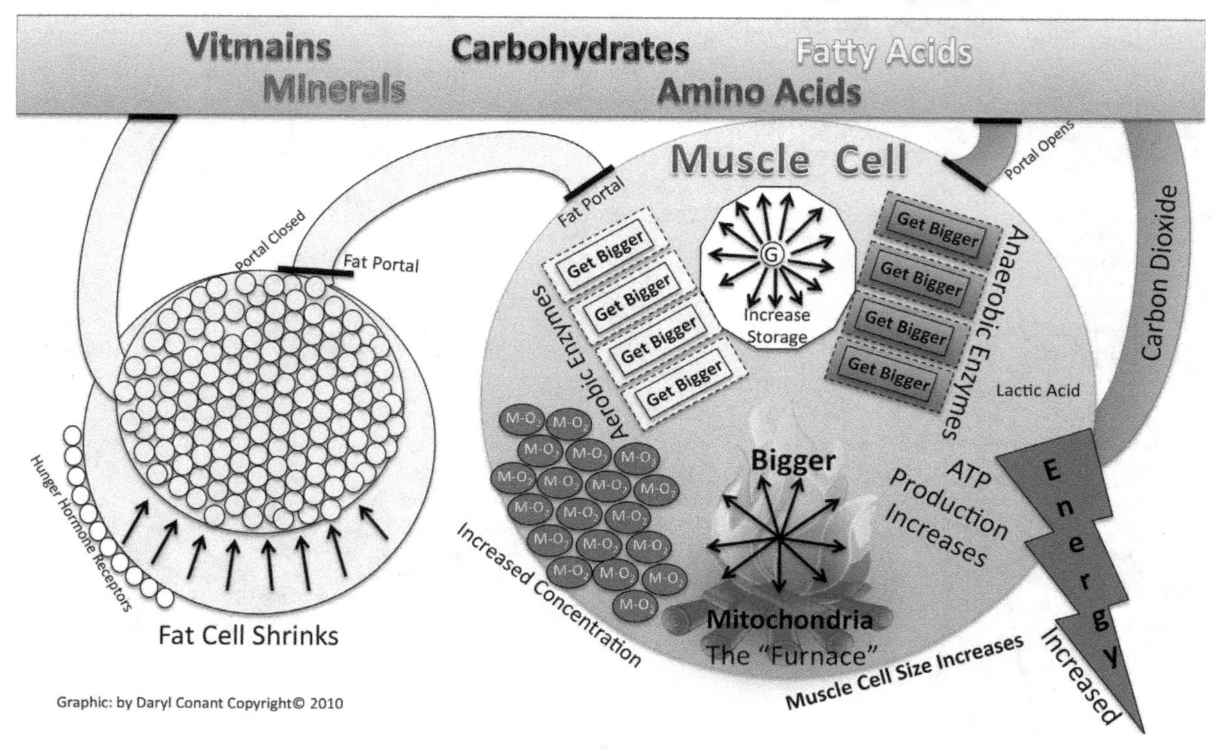


How do you increase the size of enzymes? It's simple--exercise! There are two types of metabolic processes that the muscle can use to produce energy. They are anaerobic metabolism, and aerobic metabolism. There are two phases of anaerobic metabolism that produce energy: anaerobic (without oxygen) glycolysis (phase I) and aerobic (with oxygen) glycolysis (phase II). In phase one, the muscle uses its stored glycogen (sugar) to help produce energy for a muscle contraction. The muscle can only sustain a short burst of energy due to lack of oxygen present.

# Anaerobic Muscle Metabolism

**NO OXYGEN Present: Anaerobic Glycolysis**

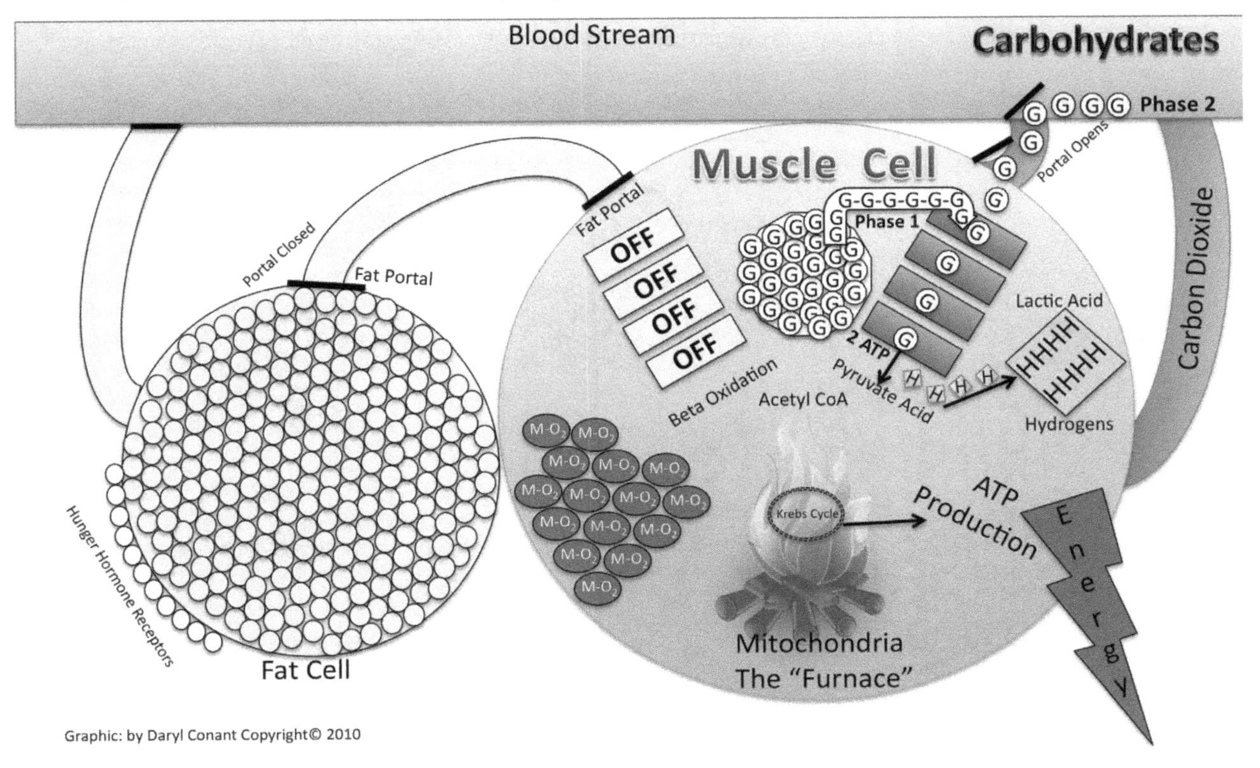


Graphic: by Daryl Conant Copyright© 2010

Phase I lasts just long enough to provide the muscle with quick bursts of energy. Sprinting fast for about a hundred yards is about how much energy Phase I provides. Phase I produces only two ATP's per glucose molecule. Once glucose gets broken down by anaerobic enzymes, the end product is pyruvate acid. Pyruvate acid yields its hydrogen ions and stores them. When there is no oxygen present, hydrogen builds up in the muscle, producing lactic acid. Lactic acid build up causes the muscle to stop contracting. The muscle needs to be replenished with oxygen in order for the lactic acid to clear.

When the duration goes longer than a few seconds, Phase II of anaerobic metabolism begins.

# Anaerobic Muscle Metabolism

**OXYGEN Present: Aerobic Glycolosis**

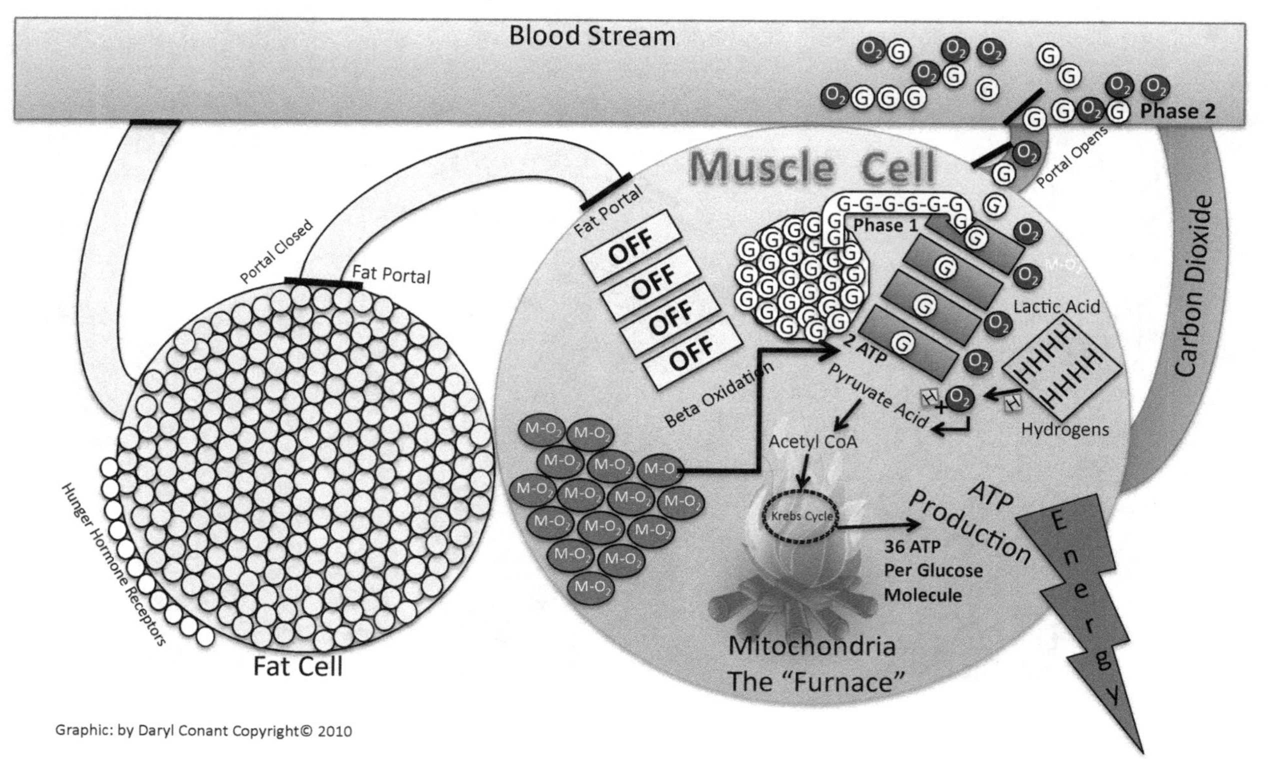


Graphic: by Daryl Conant Copyright© 2010

Phase II utilizes oxygen to help produce ATP, providing the muscle with 36 ATP per glucose molecule. Once oxygen is present it binds with hydrogen which gets converted into pyruvate acid. Pyruvate is then converted into Acetyl CoA. Acetyl CoA is an important molecule associated with aerobic metabolism. Acetyl CoA enters the Krebs cycle. The Krebs cycle, or citric acid cycle, is the end pathway of producing ATP. The end result of aerobic glycolysis is 36 ATP, providing enough energy for short, sustained exercise. Weight training and other forms of resistance training are examples of how aerobic glycolysis is used.

The sugar (anaerobic) enzymes can grow in size and take in more sugar molecules that are in the blood. This helps keep sugar from going into fat cells. Acute anaerobic exercise such as sprinting and weight lifting utilize sugar as the main source of energy. These exercises are short in duration and require little oxygen. The more sugar stored in the muscle results in greater short term bursts of high, intense energy. Eventually the glycogen levels will deplete in the muscle, forcing the muscle to build up lactic acid and ultimately shutting off the muscle. During the recovery phase, the glycogen levels are restored and the muscle is ready to respond to the short, intense exercise once it occurs again. The more intense the exercise, the greater the demand of stored sugar. The enzymes will then grow to accommodate for the new level of intensity. Having bigger sugar, burning enzymes will also help control blood sugar levels. If the active muscle tissue is depleted of glycogen then when the person eats a high carbohydrate meal, the sugar will be sucked up by the muscle cell instead of going into fat cells. Excess sugar in the blood will go into fat cells if the muscle cell is full with enough glycogen or if the muscle is inactive.

Fat metabolism is similar to sugar metabolism except that oxygen is needed to be present to help transport the fat molecules through the muscle cell.

Fat is not stored in the muscle and must be delivered from outside the cell into the cell via transporters. Transporters are amino acids that bind with the fatty acids to help the breakdown into the aerobic enzymes of the muscle cell to enter into the mitochondria for energy production. Aerobic metabolism is a bit more complex than anaerobic metabolism. For the purpose of this book, only the basic concept will be discussed.

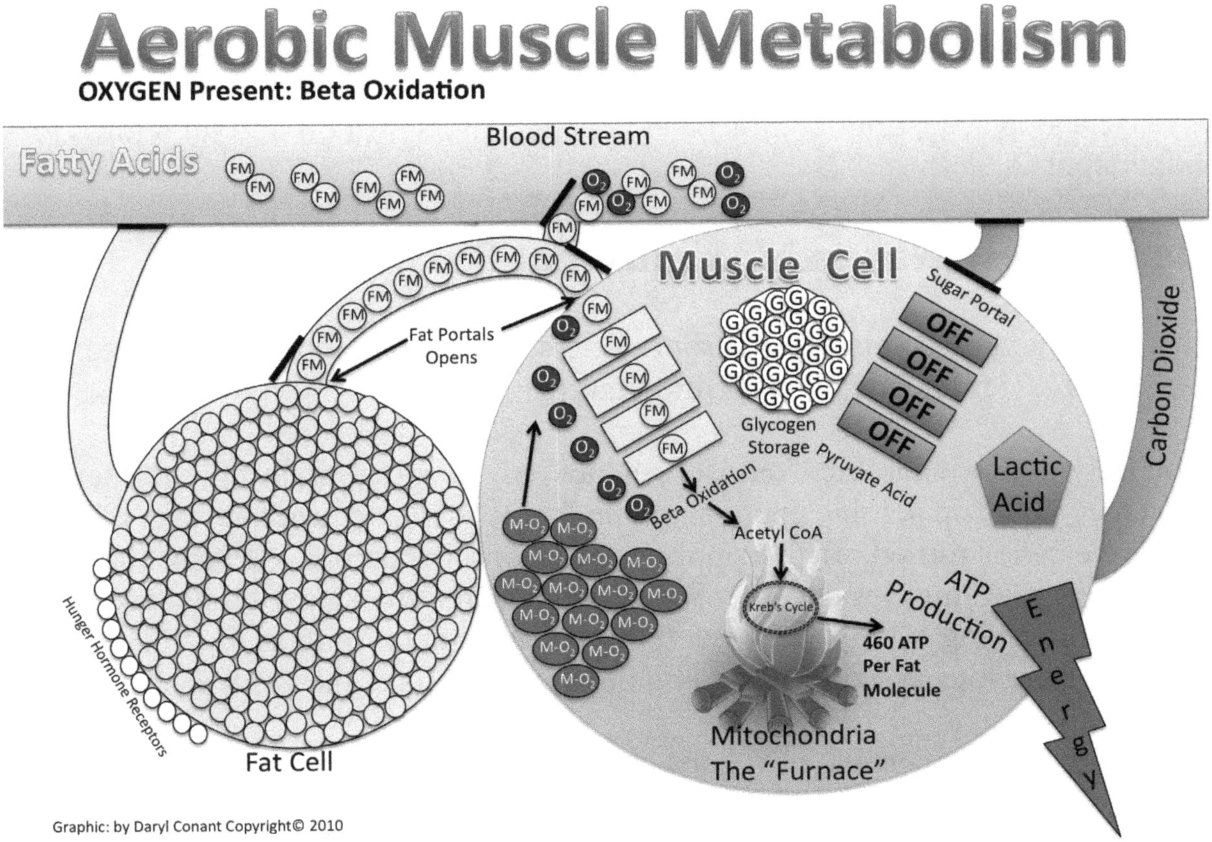

## Aerobic Muscle Metabolism

**OXYGEN Present: Beta Oxidation**

Graphic: by Daryl Conant Copyright© 2010

To transfer fatty acids from the fat cell into the muscle cell, the temperature of the muscle cell must increase. The increased heat will make the cell walls permeable for fat molecules to enter. If the muscle cell is cold or inactive, fat entry is greatly reduced. Once the muscle cell is hot enough for fat to enter, the fat molecules travel through a series of enzymatic reactions (aerobic enzymes) within the cell. Myoglobin (muscle oxygen) and blood oxygen are utilized to help assist in fatty acid delivery into the muscle cell. Through these reactions the fat molecules end up going into the mitochondrion for the production of ATP. The more muscle cells that are activated, the greater the amount of fat will be burned, resulting in greater amounts of ATP. The end result of aerobic metabolism is 460 ATP from one fat molecule. Remember, the more ATP produced the more energy the body has.

The driving force behind fat metabolism is aerobic exercise. Aerobic exercise allows oxygen to remain saturated in the muscle cell for a long duration. This is why a person can run a marathon or cycle one hundred miles; it is because they are utilizing oxygen and fat for energy. The aerobic enzymes can get bigger from frequent and sustained aerobic exercise.

Though aerobic metabolism is good for keeping a person working for long durations, the downfall is that, once you stop exercising, the aerobic enzymes in the muscle stop accepting fat molecules. The receptors turn off and fat returns to the fat depots.

## The Greatest Way to Maximize Fat Burning

In order to maximize your efforts from exercise it is important to incorporate both anaerobic and aerobic metabolism into your plan.

If you only perform aerobic exercise, you are only burning fat during the exercise bout. Once you stop aerobic exercising, the fat molecules return to the fat cells and the muscle cell is turned off. The more you perform the aerobic exercise the more conditioned your muscles become. When you become fitter your body becomes better at conserving energy. So, essentially you are not burning as much fat because the nervous system has figured out a way to make the work easier.

To burn a higher percentage of fat, the muscle cell has to be influenced by greater intensity--*resistance training*. Incorporating resistance training (weight training, sprinting) can influence greater fat burning than just performing aerobic exercise alone. The main source of energy for resistance training is sugar. Fat metabolism is reduced dramatically during intense exercise. However, once your blood pressure and heart rate comes down from the intense exercise, your body enters into the "thermogenic effect," which proves that resistance training is the greatest fat burner of all.

Remember the thermogenic effect is the process by which the body generates heat, or energy, by increasing the metabolic rate above normal. The longer the thermogenic effect lasts the more effective fat burning becomes. During high intense exercise, such as weight lifting, the body reaches high levels of muscular heat. The muscles are pumped up with blood causing an increase in muscle metabolism. During weight training the main fuel supply is sugar.

However, once the exercise session ends and tissue repair begins, fat metabolism turns on. I believe that the reason for the increased release of fat from the fat stores is to help cool down the muscle tissue. Heat allows fat to be reduced into liquid form making it easier to oxidize in the muscle cell. Through the process of oxidation the muscle cell cools down. This is known as paying back the oxygen debt. Also, the fat soluble vitamins (A, D, E, K) found in fat help replenish and repair damaged muscle tissue. Fat is necessary for the production of muscle tissue and it helps cool down the muscle tissue back to the resting metabolic rate.

To maximize the thermogenic effect, the exercise intensity must be high enough to create a *metabolic boost*. The metabolic boost is a shift in energy and heat production of the muscle tissue. Though resistance training is the best for burning overall fat percentages, aerobic exercise is still important in the overall development of muscle cells and the health of all the systems of the body.

The benefits of muscle metabolism as a result of both aerobic and anaerobic exercise are: fat cells shrink, aerobic and anaerobic enzymes get bigger, myoglobin concentrations in oxidative muscle cells increase in concentration, the number and size of mitochondria increase, muscle glycogen stores increase, improved lactate levels and increased energy.

# Nutrients: The Basis Of Life

Vitamins, Minerals, Protein, Fat, Carbohydrates, Water, Fiber

## Vitamins:

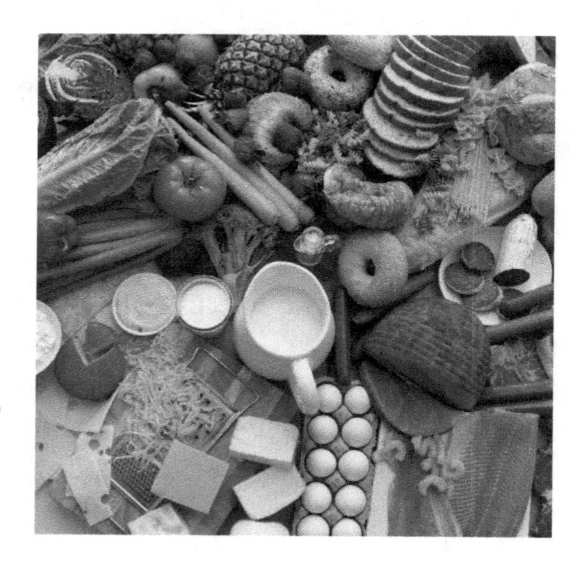

Vitamins are found in all living things and are essential for the body. Most vitamins have to come from external sources with the exception of a few, which are non essential. There are two groups of vitamins: ***water soluble and fat soluble.***

Vitamins B, C, and bioflavonoids, are water soluble. Water soluble means that they absorb in water and are transported within the intracellular fluid of the cell. Water soluble vitamins have to be replenished frequently throughout the diet because they get flushed out of the body everyday. When the body eliminates urine, both Vitamins B and C are reduced in the body and must be replenished from food sources. The fat soluble vitamins (A, D, E, K) are more stable in the body and are stored in body fat. Fat helps deliver fat soluble vitamins throughout the cells of the body. Fat soluble vitamins are rarely depleted from the body, and do not need to replaced every day like water soluble vitamins do.

The way vitamins work is that they are reactive with enzymes (catalyst's). Oxidation is the primary role for enzymes in the body. A protein molecule and a co-enzyme make up an enzyme. Enzymes are the catalyst for all cellular chemical reactions. Co-enzymes are vitamins that interact with a protein molecule to initiate a cellular reaction. This reaction sequence occurs a thousand times a day, supplying the cells with proper nutrient support. When there is a vitamin deficiency, the cells suffer and the body becomes malnourished. Consuming foods rich in vitamins will help ensure proper nutrition to the cells to keep the body systems working efficiently.

The following is only a brief description of the essential vitamins the body requires. If you want to learn more about vitamins, I suggest you seek further learning available in libraries and book stores. They are many in number and many are very detailed.

***Vitamin A***

Vitamin A (carotene) is a fat soluble vitamin that helps aid in the growth and repair of body tissues. It helps protect skin, and defends the membranes of the mouth, nose, throat and lungs against infection. Carotene is found in; eggs, carrots, green leafy vegetables, and fish and animal fat. Fish oil is a supplement that has a rich supply of carotene.
***Recommended daily allowance: 600 µg***

***Vitamin B Complex***

Vitamin B Complex is water soluble: B1 (thiamine), B2 (riboflavin), B3 (niacin), B5 (pantothenic acid), B6 (pyridoxine), B12 (cyanobalamin), B15 (panagamic acid), biotin, choline, folic acid, inositol, and PABA (para-aminodbenzoic acid). Vitamin B complex plays a major role in cellular metabolism. Carbohydrates are converted into glucose with the use of vitamin B complex, as well as fat and protein metabolism. The greatest attribute that Vitamin B complex has to offer is how it nourishes the nervous system. Psychological well-being is dependent on the Vitamin B complex. Many psychological disorders are nutrient-related and a poor supply of the Vitamin B complex can contribute to nervous system dysfunction. Food sources of Vitamin B include: eggs, whole grains, poultry, green vegetables, fish, fruits, milk, and brewer's yeast. Brewer's yeast is the richest source of vitamin B complex. Excessive use of alcohol and caffeine can have an adverse effect on folic acid and thiamine, resulting in the disruption of healthy nervous system function. ***Recommended daily allowance:*** $B_1$***-1.4mg,*** $B_2$***-1.6mg,*** $B_3$***-18 mg,*** $B_5$***-6 mg,*** $B_6$***-2mg,*** $B_{12}$***-6µg***

***Vitamin C***

Known as ascorbic acid, Vitamin C is a crucial water soluble vitamin that is unstable. Heat, light, oxidation, and oxygen can destroy Vitamin C. Vitamin C is vital in keeping the immune system free of radical invaders. Vitamin C helps with the formation of collagen for connective tissue found in skin, bone, and ligaments. Stress to the body burns up vitamin C rapidly. Vitamin C must be consumed regularly to sustain its value in the body. A diet low in Vitamin C will result in a body that is more susceptible to infection or illness. Good sources of Vitamin C are: citrus fruits, tomatoes, and green vegetables. ***Recommended daily allowance: 75 mg-100 mg***

***Vitamin D***

Vitamin D is a fat-soluble substance. It is the only vitamin that can be derived by food or sunlight. Bone and teeth development are dependent on vitamin D. Vitamin D works synergistically with calcium to provide optimal function of calcium ions for cellular metabolism. Sources of Vitamin D are: milk, fish, egg yolks, chicken liver, and direct sunlight. ***Recommended daily allowance:*** **5**µg

***Vitamin E***

Vitamin E is a fat-soluble vitamin that is an anti-oxidant it protects the blood stream from harmful invaders. Vitamin E plays a major role in the cellular respiration of all muscles, cardiac and skeletal. Oxidation of cells increases the aging process and since Vitamin E helps reduce oxidation and it slows down the aging process. Vitamin E is highly necessary for strength and endurance. The best sources of Vitamin E are; wheat germ, vegetable oils, whole raw seeds and nuts, and soybeans. ***Recommended daily allowance: 10 mg***

***Vitamin K***

Vitamin K is a fat-soluble vitamin that is produced in the intestines. Low carbohydrates and high protein diets tend to increase the formation of Vitamin K in the intestines. Vitamin K is produced by the flora in the intestines. It helps with the formation of good bacteria. If the flora are compromised, then Vitamin K can be depleted and bad bacteria can take over the intestines. Aspirin, radiation, pharmaceutical drugs, antibiotics, and rancid fats all destroy Vitamin K. Deficiencies of Vitamin K are rare, therefore, supplementation of Vitamin K is not necessary. The best sources of Vitamin K are: kelp, alfalfa, green leafy vegetables, cow's milk, yogurt, egg yolks, molasses, safflower oil, and polyunsaturated oils. ***Recommended daily allowance: 80*** µg

## Minerals

Minerals are essential for proper functioning of all cells in the body. Sodium, calcium, magnesium, phosphorus, iron, iodine, potassium, zinc and manganese are the main minerals that the body utilizes for cellular respiration and metabolism. The cells also use trace minerals copper, selenium, cobalt and chromium.

### *Sodium*

Sodium works in opposition to potassium ions; thus creating an electrostatic charge on a cell. A voltage change occurs by reaction of the nerve impulses. Too much sodium in the body causes problems with the electrical conductivity of the nerve impulses which can cause health problems or even death. Though sodium is essential for the health of the body, too much can wreak havoc. Most foods contain a certain amount of sodium. As long as the foods are low in sodium the need to ever add sodium to food should not be considered.

### *Calcium*

Calcium plays an important role in cellular electrical conductivity of muscle and nerve cells. The body cannot manufacture calcium, and so it must be derived from diet. Excess calcium in the body is stored in bone. Low levels of calcium can result in bone and tooth loss and poor conductivity of muscles; i.e. heart. Calcium is an essential mineral found in: dairy products, kale, kelp, broccoli, oranges, almonds, green peas, spinach, baked beans and black beans.
***Recommended daily allowance: 1000 mg***

### *Magnesium*

Magnesium is the second most concentrated mineral in the body,calcium being the first. The role of magnesium is to help with energy production in cells (ATP production). It helps with the formation of proteins and is the antagonist against calcium to help restore muscle contractions. Magnesium is also used to balance the sodium/potassium pump within cells. It is important in hormone production. It also helps reduce excess levels of calcium in the blood and helps prevent kidney stones. Deficiencies in magnesium can result in high blood pressure, poor circulation, involuntary muscle twitches, anaemia, anxiety, menstrual cramps, muscle cramps, and sugar cravings. Magnesium absorption can be affected by excessive alcohol consumption, irritable digestive tract, and high calcium concentrations. Sources of magnesium include kelp, wheat bran, wheat germ, almonds, cashews, molasses, buckwheat, hazelnuts, roasted peanuts, dried apricots, avocado, parsley, sunflower seeds, garlic, broccoli, cheddar cheese, cauliflower, celery, chicken, beef, asparagus, tomatoes, eggs, and whole milk. ***Recommended daily allowance: 5 mg***

***Phosphorus***

Phosphorus is an essential component of bones and teeth and is required to activate B-complex vitamins. It makes up the cytoplasm of the cell. It is a major contributor in the function of many enzymes, energy production (ATP) and cell division. Deficiency in phosphorus can be result in poor energy production in the body. Good sources of phosphorus are nuts, meat, fish, cheese, soy products and whole grains. ***Recommended daily allowance: 1000 mg***

***Iron***

Iron is the main component of hemoglobin, which helps in the transportation of oxygen and carbon dioxide to and from the lungs. It plays a role in enzyme and energy production. Iron is an antioxidant that helps clear out free radicals that invade the body and helps boost the immune system. Deficiencies in iron can be related to; anemia, chronic fatigue, pale skin, irrational sleep patterns, restless leg syndrome, lack of attention, learning difficulties, breathlessness, body temperature fluctuations, frequent infections, and some types of deafness. Sources of iron are, kelp, curry powder, brewers yeast, some breakfast cereals, molasses, wheat germ, soy flour, sunflower seeds, parsley, clams, almonds, dried apricots, cashews, tomato puree, beef liver, meat, eggs, broccoli, olives, peanuts, walnuts, and green peas.

***Recommended daily allowance: 15 mg***

***Iodine***

Iodine is required for the production of thyroxine. Thyroxine is the hormone produced by the thyroid gland and is essential in controlling the metabolic rate. Iodine helps with the development of the fetal nervous system and is important for the development of healthy connective tissue. It also helps with the regulation of estrogen in breast tissue. Deficiencies in iodine can result in dry skin, excessive estrogen production, hypothyroidism, chronic fatigue, reduced immune system function, and goiter (increased thyroid gland). Sources of iodine include: broccoli, cabbage, kale, lima beans, mustard, peanuts, and sweet potato.

***Recommended daily allowance: 150 µg***

***Potassium***

Potassium is an important mineral that helps to oppose sodium and influence cell polarization. It regulates heart function, regulates blood pressure, protein synthesis, nerve conduction, converts glucose into muscle glycogen (sugar), regulates balance function in the kidneys and is essential in carbon dioxide elimination. It also

maintains acid and alkaline pH balance and balances muscle contractibility. Deficiencies in potassium could result in electrolyte imbalances, affecting muscle contractibility and nerve conductivity. Other problems include dehydration, heart contraction irregularity, and poor kidney function. This mineral is usually reduced dramatically during times of illness when body fluids are eliminated in abnormal amounts (diarrhea, vomiting and excessive sweating). It is important to maintain proper levels of electrolytes throughout the day. Sources of potassium are bananas, avocados, potatoes, raisins, salmon, whole milk, chicken, dried apricots, tomatoes, lima beans (cooked), and cauliflower.
***Recommended daily allowance: 1000 mg***

***Zinc***
When the immune system is compromised and a cold develops, we are told to take zinc and vitamin C. Zinc boosts the immune system to keep it strong. Zinc is also important for hundreds of biological enzymatic reactions in the body, such as sperm production, ovulation, and fertilization. Zinc is an antioxidant that contributes to good skin health. Deficiencies in zinc can result in reproductive dysfunction, digestive problems, and reduced immune production. Sources of zinc are beef, lamb, pork, turkey, chicken, clams, salmon, milk, cheese, yeast, peanuts, beans, whole grain cereals, brown rice, potatoes, and yogurt.
***Recommended daily allowance: 15 mg***

***Manganese***
Manganese is an important trace mineral that is found in the liver, kidney, pancreas, skin, muscles, and bones. Manganese plays a major role in the development of bone and the thyroid hormone, thyroxine. Deficiencies in manganese can include the development of diabetes, weak bones, failing memory, dizziness, and poor muscle coordination. Sources of manganese are all green leafy vegetables, beans, whole grains, nuts, and egg yolks.
***Recommended daily allowance: 5 mg***

When taking a mineral supplement it is best to consume chelated minerals. Minerals are known as being chelated when amino acids (proteins) attach themselves around the mineral. This protective coating helps with the transport of the tablet through the digestive system. The coating value differs with different products. The cheaper types tend to be poor in value, where as the more expensive types absorb better. If the tablet has a poor coating when it enters into the stomach acid, it will break down too quickly. The mineral is then prematurely released and will no longer be available to enter into the bloodstream. When a capsule enters into the stomach it is broken down by hydrochloric acid (HCL) within a couple of minutes. A tablet takes longer, about fifteen minutes, to break down. During the time of digestive breakdown the chelated coating breaks off making the mineral vulnerable to attachment to anything in its vicinity. This could cause the mineral not to make it to the small intestines for absorption.

The best approach is to purchase supplements that are chelated with a pH sensitive amino acid coating of milk solids rather than amino acids from vegetable proteins. Vegetable proteins break down faster, making the mineral less likely to be absorbed into the bloodstream. Be careful with ingesting cheap mineral products. Cheap minerals provide no value. Due to acid rain and other pollutants that have spread on the Earth, natural organic minerals are becoming harder to obtain through food sources. I recommend taking a daily mineral complex supplement to help ensure proper mineral intake each day.

## Water

Water is the most important nutrient of the body. A person can only live two to ten days without water, depending on temperature and how much you weigh. The human body is made up of seventy percent water. Water is the main component in all cells. It is important to drink clean, non-chlorinated water and to drink small amounts of water throughout the day. It is best not to guzzle water, rather, you should drink it in small quantities more frequently throughout the day. Guzzling down a huge glass of water will be counterproductive. Unfortunately, in this day and age our water supply is tainted with chemicals. Much of the municipal water supply is mixed with chlorine and other agents to kill off bacteria and metals that are leached into the water supply. It is a shame that you can't drink water from a faucet without ingesting chemicals. We have to resort to purchasing water filters or bottled water. Chlorine is a dangerous chemical that can destroy the thyroid gland in humans. Taking a shower without a water filter also allows chlorinated water to get into your body. Years of taking showers using municipal water or swimming in chlorinated pools increases the risk for developing thyroid complications.

The skin is permeable by nature and chlorine and other agents can be absorbed through the skin. The best way to safeguard yourself against the toxic levels of chlorine is to use water filters for drinking and bathing and to drink bottled water from reliable companies. If you can't get clean water, you can drink distilled water. Distilled water doesn't have the mineral content of regular water but it is free of chlorine and other toxic chemicals.

# Protein

Protein is the most important food source for the body. Hippocrates concluded 2500 years ago that protein is the most important nutrient for proper human development and life. All living cells are comprised of protein. Protein is the building material of life. Muscle, organs, bones, cartilage, skin, antibodies, some hormones, all enzymes, the compounds that direct chemical reactions in cells, are made of proteins. From the moment of conception, protein is constantly working to build new cells for growth. Throughout our lifespan the cells of our body are constantly dying and reproducing. Cellular replication depends on protein. Protein is broken down into amino acids, which are known as the building blocks. There are two subtypes of amino acids: *essential* and *non-essential.* Non essential are the amino acids that our body can produce on its own. Essential amino acids are not produced by our body and must come from external sources.

Plant and animal sources supply the required essential amino acids for proper nutrition. The best source of protein comes from animal sources. Animal protein contains all the essential amino acids. Vegetables, on the other hand, contain incomplete proteins. For example, red beans are an incomplete protein; however, when mixed with rice all the essential aminos are derived. It is harder for vegetarians to get all the essential amino acids into their diet than those that eat meat, cheese, dairy and eggs.

When we eat foods containing protein, the digestive system breaks it down into the constituent amino acids. These then enter the body "pool" of amino acids. Each cell then assembles the proteins it needs using the building blocks (amino acids) available. If, however, one or more of the needed amino acids is in short supply or not available at all, the other amino acids that may be on hand cannot be utilized from a protein. This is why it is important to eat a diet that contains all of the essential amino acids, plus enough additional amino acids to allow for synthesis of the non-essential amino acids.

When a person doesn't take in enough dietary protein, the body will utilize its own muscle protein to supply the immune system and vital organs. ***The appropriate amount of dietary protein is as follows: sedentary adult .8 x body weight (BW) = Daily Required Intake (DRI), active adult 1 x BW = DRI, Athlete 1.2 x BW= DRI. The result is how many grams of protein you should consume daily.***

Sources of protein are beef, poultry, fish, eggs, dairy products, nuts, seeds, and legumes like black beans and lentils.

# Fiber

Fiber is overrated. We have been taught by doctors to eat a tremendous amount of fiber throughout the day. Many people who suffer from elimination problems are told to increase their fiber intake. The reason for their elimination problems could be due to the fact that they are eating valueless food, compromising the digestive system. Eating too much fiber can actually be bad for the digestive system. Too much fiber can clear out the good bacteria in the intestines. Having good bacteria in the intestines is essential for good health. Eating fresh fruits and vegetables on a daily basis will promote proper elimination and provide you with enough dietary fiber. There is plenty of fiber in vegetables and fruits to suffice without having to add additional fiber to the diet. If you adhere to a healthy nutrition plan and still have elimination issues it is advised that you consult your primary care doctor for help.

# Fat

Over the past twenty-five years, Americans have been forced to believe that fat and cholesterol should not be consumed. Crazy marketing schemes and absurd diets have been devised that take out all fats and cholesterol from foods. We have bought into the idea that if we cut out all cholesterol and fats from our diet, our blood cholesterol levels will drop. This is just not true. Did you know that if you take away external sources of cholesterol and fats from the diet your body will actually produce more cholesterol internally? The way this works is that the liver is constantly breaking down fats, proteins and sugars preparing these substrates to enter the bloodstream. This regulatory system is governed by the needs of all the internal organs. If the body is not getting the correct amount of dietary cholesterol through digestion, then the blood stream is disrupted and threatened from being cholesterol deficient. The liver remedies the threat by producing more cholesterol. Often times more cholesterol is produced by the body to help prevent against deprivation. Cholesterol is important to the blood and the cells of the body and more is produced if there is a deficiency. Without it the cells and hormone production begin to suffer. Cholesterol is essential for building and repairing the body. Cholesterol is found in the cell membranes to help with permeability and substrate exchange. Cholesterol also helps with hormone activity in the body. DHEA (dihydroepiandersterone), progesterone, testosterone, estradiol, cortisol and Vitamin D are developed in the body with cholesterol being the main constituent. When the body is deficient in cholesterol, the body is compromised, altering the cell growth. Catabolic aging is increased and cell replication slows down considerably. Cholesterol plays a big part in the health of the nervous system and brain function. All the nerves are insulated by cholesterol.

Fat is labeled as an evil food. Again, the media teaches us that if you eat fat you will become fat. This is ridiculous! In order for fat to be stored in the body, insulin must be released from the pancreas to drive fat into fat cells. When you ingest dietary fat into your body insulin remains stable and is not released from the pancreas. Fat cells will remain closed and will not take in fat. Another key point is that when you eat dietary fat the liver has to work to breakdown the fat to prepare it to enter into the bloodstream. The liver is devised of complex enzymes that break down foods used by the body. When too much of something in ingested by the body, the liver will pull more water into itself to help break the substance down. If there is still a dangerous level of a substance trying to get into the body, the liver will force the body to purge it out. By the time fat gets into the bloodstream the quantity is not as much as you may think. The liver is the filter and the regulator: it is a remarkable organ and system. The body is designed to emulsify fat and cholesterol. When you eat a diet that has healthy fats in it, you will have sustained energy for hours because fat becomes the main fuel source. There are nine calories to every gram of fat, whereas protein and carbohydrates have only four calories per one gram. What this means is that fat is a better energy sustainer.

Carbohydrates burn out faster and have to constantly be replenished, where as fat sustains energy for hours. This is why so many people get addicted to sugar, their bloodstream doesn't want all the excess sugar in the body so it is always in a battle to clear it out into the liver, muscle, or fat cells. Dietary fat not only helps fuel the body, it helps influence the release of stored fat.

Fat is essential for transporting vitamins, insulating the body, providing energy and helping to cushion joints. When the body is deprived of dietary fat, the body is compromised, thus making the release of stored fat difficult. In fact, not eating enough dietary fat can increase the likelihood that a person will suffer from; increased carbohydrate cravings, constipation, thinning hair, infertility, insomnia, loss of lean body mass, increase of abdominal, buttock and thigh fat, psychological disorders, and skin problems.

Dietary fat is essential for good health and should be considered an important part of your nutrition program.

## Good Sources of Fat

Is it possible to overeat healthy fats? Yes! However, the body has a built in feedback system that will be alerted when too much fat is ingested. The stomach will not be able to sustain proper breakdown of the fats which will cause an ill feeling, and in some cases vomiting is the result.

Fats are comprised of fatty acids. Fatty acids are made up of long chains of carbon molecules that are bound together. The molecular chain has four sides of carbon attached to itself. There are two carbons molecules attached to each other while the other two sides are unbonded. The unbonded sides are filled with hydrogen atoms, forming what are known as **saturated fats.** Saturated fats are formed as solid fat. Butter, lard, types of animal fat, cream, and eggs are examples of saturated fat. Saturated fats such as butter and eggs are best for cooking.

If there is an absent hydrogen atom in the carbon molecular chain then the fat becomes less dense, forming what is known as **monounsaturated fats.** The more the carbon molecular chain lacks hydrogen atoms the more liquid the fat becomes forming **polyunsaturated fats.** Types of monounsaturated fats and polyunsaturated fats are olive oil, safflower oil, peanut oil, fish oils, and nuts. Monounsaturated fats and polyunsaturated fats are not recommended for cooking.

The controversy about fats stems from eating saturated fats, monounsaturated fats, and polyunsaturated fats. We believe that we should avoid eating all saturated fats and eat more of the mono and polyunsaturated fats. This is not true. All three types of fats are healthy and important for normal functioning of the body. The body is designed to metabolize these fats with ease. Meat fat (saturated) has been digested by the human body for thousands of years, as I mentioned earlier. There is a big misconception when it comes to eating saturated fats. It has been suggested that if you eat meat, that your internal blood cholesterol will increase and you will die of a heart attack. I disagree with this! I believe that the body is designed to digest saturated fats and that we should eat them as a part of a balanced nutrition plan.

There are circumstances when eating fat is bad for you. Eating damaged fats that have been tampered with either by processing or being overcooked, can contribute to heart disease, illness, and internal arterial damage. Damaged fats such as hydrogenated fats, trans-fatty acids, and oxidized fats are bad for you and should be avoided. Untampered saturated fat is not the the problem, damaged fats are. Damaged fats contribute to a wide variety health issues in humans.

**Hydrogenated fats** are fats that have been tampered with. Too many hydrogen atoms become attached to the carbon molecular chain causing an extremely tight bond, so tight that the body cannot recognize the configuration and cannot break them down. This forms free radicals in the blood. If too many of these free radical fatty acids form they can clog up arteries.

**Oxidized fats** are fats that have become rancid. When healthy fats are exposed to air, the electron balance of the fat is displaced and this forms into a damaged fat. Oils that are left out in room temperature can very easily become rancid and should not be ingested. Be sure to refrigerate fats and look at the expiration date before consuming.

**Trans-fatty acids** are polyunsaturated fats that are processed and taken out of their natural molecular configuration. As I mentioned earlier, polyunsaturated fats are healthy fats. What makes polyunsaturated fats good is that the carbon and hydrogen atoms are configured correctly to form a desirable fat. Polyunsaturated fats are unstable if they are tampered with. The carbon and hydrogen bonds become unstable. The hydrogen atoms get transferred to the opposite side of the carbon atoms, thus making the fat too difficult for the body to metabolize. Free radicals enter into the bloodstream and can cause havoc to the arteries. Many of the foods that Americans consume are loaded with trans-fatty acids.

Polyunsaturated fats are good to ingest if taken in their natural, raw form, i.e.: seeds, nuts, fish. Never cook with polyunsaturated oils. The heat damages the carbon and hydrogen bonds and makes the oil bad which will get into the food that is cooked, producing free radical formation in the blood when ingested.

## How to Eat Fat

Try to eat fat in its natural state.

- Avoid over cooking animal products, as this damages the carbon and hydrogen bonds of fat.

- Man made processed fats should be avoided. Remember that all natural food has all the active enzymes and healthy fats intact. Cooking or processing these live active enzymes will destroy them. In fact just about everything man made should be avoided. Natural food is the best way go.

- Keep fats in a cool dry place in order to avoid rancidity.
- Always mix a protein with a non-damaged fat. Avoid eliminating all fat when eating a protein. Protein must be accompanied by fat to hydrolyze through the liver.

- Eliminate partially hydrogenated and completely hydrogenated oils from your diet.

- Cook meat just enough to kill off any bacteria. Middle should be red and juicy, not dry or burnt.

- Don't be afraid to eat non-tampered saturated and poly-unsaturated fats.

- Eat nitrate-free fats.

- Eating fats within the correct amounts is healthy. Avoid over consuming fats.

- Eat eggs that are from free range chickens that are not corn fed. Find eggs that have a rich omega 3 content. Also rich in Omega 3 are olive oil, avocados, dark green leafy vegetables, salmon, flax seed oil, walnut oil, nuts, fish, ostrich, grass fed beef bison, and game meats.

- Omega 6 fats are essential for health. However, avoid over consuming them as this can lead to overproduction of inflammation-producing prostaglandins (PGE2s, PGE1s and PGE2s), which can lead to health problems. Vegetable oils and non-grass fed animal products contain higher levels of omega 6 fats than animal sources that are organically regulated. Consume sparingly.

**Sources of polyunsaturated fats**: liquid oils, corn oil, safflower oil, sesame oil, sunflower oil, walnut oil, soybean oil, poppyseed oil, salmon oil, flaxseed oil, wheat germ oil, and primrose oil.

**Sources of monounsaturated fats** almond oil, avocado oil, grape-seed oil, olive oil, hazelnut oil and rice oil.

**Sources of saturated fats:** butter, cheese, chicken fat, cream, duck fat, eggs, sour cream, and turkey fat.

# Is Eating Cholesterol Good For You!

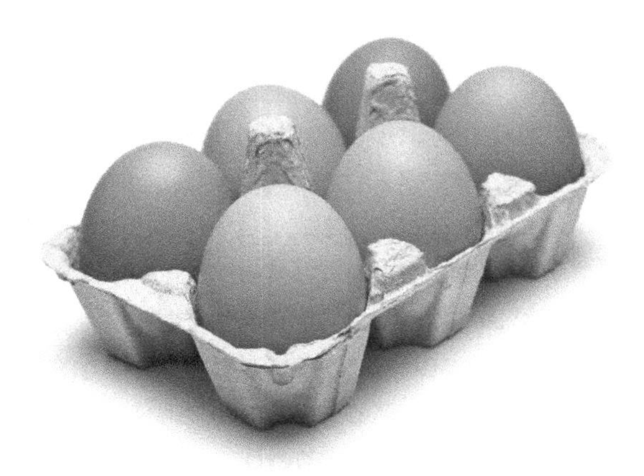

I don't care what the doctors say. I disagree with the low-fat diet plan. Telling someone to avoid eating cholesterol and to eat more carbohydrates is ludicrous to me. The problem with eating carbohydrates in excess is that the liver cannot handle the high influx of sugar. The liver then must convert the sugar into triglycerides, cholesterol or glycogen, depending on what the need may be.

When sugar is consumed it goes through the small intestine and enters the portal vein. Insulin is released to help deliver the sugar to the cells. Then sugar goes to the liver. The liver decides if the amount is satisfactory enough to enter the bloodstream. If too much sugar is coming into the liver then the liver breaks it down. The reason for this is to prevent the brain from receiving too much sugar. A little sugar is fine but too much is dangerous.

The liver will only use the sugar for energy and glycogen storage if there is a need for it. If liver glycogen levels are full in the liver and muscles and there is no immediate energy need, then the liver will convert the sugar into cholesterol or triglycerides.

Cutting out cholesterol from your diet will put the blood and VNES system into a defensive state. External cholesterol deprivation causes a series of cascading events that contribute to the increase of internal cholesterol production. High carbohydrate and low cholesterol levels in the blood signal the sugar radar releasing insulin, which in, turn activates the release of an enzyme in the liver known as HMG CO-A Reductose. This enzyme is responsible for over-producing cholesterol in the blood. When sugars are high in the blood stream the liver will use up the available sugar and continue to produce internal cholesterol. Sugar molecules activate the production of HMG CO-A Reductose. In order to turn off the HMG CO-A Reductose enzyme healthy external dietary cholesterol must be present. High carbohydrate and low-fat diets will always activate the sugar radar response.

There are medications prescribed by doctors that reduce internal cholesterol. Physicians prescribe statin-type drugs (Lipitor) to block the HMG CO-A Reductose enzyme. But rather than telling their patient to eat healthy cholesterol, they tell their patient to eat a low-fat, high-carbohydrate diet and avoid cholesterol altogether. This becomes dangerous, because even though the statin drug stops the production of internal cholesterol, insulin is still responding to the high sugar content. Their cholesterol levels may drop but it is only because of the blocking effect of the statin drug. Blocking one enzyme doesn't shut off the entire sequence; the liver, heart and blood system are still at risk of developing disease from not having enough good dietary cholesterol. One of the best natural ways to safe guard from developing high internal cholesterol is to eat good dietary cholesterol.

Whenever the bloodstream is dealing with high sugar and insulin levels, cholesterol is constantly being produced. A person can be on a low-fat diet and still have very high internal cholesterol levels. Stress, caffeine, alcohol, tobacco, aspartame, sedentary living, stimulants, some medications, and a low-fat diet will all increase insulin levels and cause inflammatory effects in the body.

Low-fat, high-carbohydrate diets will over produce internal cholesterol levels and promote the risk of having a stroke, developing heart disease, or developing the onset of arteriolosclerosis. Healthy fats are essential for good health.

## Cholesterol and Exercise

Cholesterol helps repair damaged tissue. Exercise breaks down muscle tissue in the body. How much muscle breakdown that occurs is dependent on how intense the exercise is. Weight training can produce a lot of muscle breakdown if the intensities are great enough. The breakdown of muscle tissue is a normal effect from weight training. With proper recovery and nutritional support, the body rebuilds the damaged tissue building more muscle tissue.

Whenever the tissue is damaged, cholesterol, is released to help repair the tissue. During the break down of muscle, sugar is released into the bloodstream, which causes a slight elevation in blood cholesterol levels, which is normal. The cholesterol is needed to help re-establish muscle protein synthesis. High density lipoprotein (HDL) levels increase as a result of exercise. The greater the exercise intensity the more damage occurs, and therefore more cholesterol is produced.

# Food Combining

I am a firm believer that the body is designed to metabolize protein and complex carbohydrates separately. Fruits should be eaten by themselves, never to be mixed with proteins. Proteins should be eaten by themselves or with a water soluble vegetable. When protein is being digested, the intestines pulls in water to help aid in digestion, making protein a dehydrating factor. The same holds true for complex carbohydrates. Like protein, carbohydrates pull water into the intestines to assist in digestion, making it also a dehydrating factor. When you combine both a protein and a complex carbohydrate into the digestive system, too much water is pulled in. There is not enough water to help with the digestive properties to break down both complex compounds. The result is poor digestion. Fermentation develops when food stay in the digestive tract for too long. When foods become difficult to breakdown they sit in the intestines, eventually spoiling. Fermentation produces an uncomfortable bloated feeling that often produces severe gas pains.

Proteins digest in an acid-based medium. Carbohydrates digest in an alkaline-based medium. When both a protein and a complex carbohydrate are combined, the acid and alkaline digestive enzymes mix together, causing fermentation and toxic by-products that put a strain on the digestive system. During times of digestive stress, stress hormones are released to help get rid of the dangerous mixture. Cortisol inhibits nutrient uptake through the intestinal walls. The food is eliminated through the bowels. When the nutrients are not absorbed through the intestines, the body goes into a catabolic state. This can lead to high blood pressure, high cholesterol, carbohydrate cravings, fatigue, illness, and immune system suppression. This is why it is important to eat water soluble vegetables with concentrated proteins and concentrated carbohydrates. The water from the vegetables helps aid in digestion. Concentrated proteins and carbohydrates should not be combined at the same time.

It is important to follow the correct methods of eating to keep the digestive system healthy. Poor food combinations will wreak havoc on the body's vital nutrient exchange system (VNES). I believe that many digestive illnesses are a result of poor dietary food combinations. The human being is designed to eat one type of food at a time. It is not designed to consume large quantities of different types of food at one time. When we overeat and combine too many types of food it can result in: gas; bloating; fatigue; diarrhea; dehydration; muscle weakness; dizziness; nausea; increased blood pressure; allergies; low blood sugar; headaches;

constipation, and illness. The following is a chart outlining the rules of food combining. Protein and starches are a poor combination. Concentrated protein foods should not be combined with other fats. Concentrated protein already has concentrated fat mixed with it. Adding more fats changes the molecular configurations of the concentrated proteins making it harder to digest. Fats and starches can be combined without compromising the system. Non-starchy vegetables and starches can be mixed safely. Proteins and non-starchy vegetables are a good combination. Fruits should be eaten by themselves.

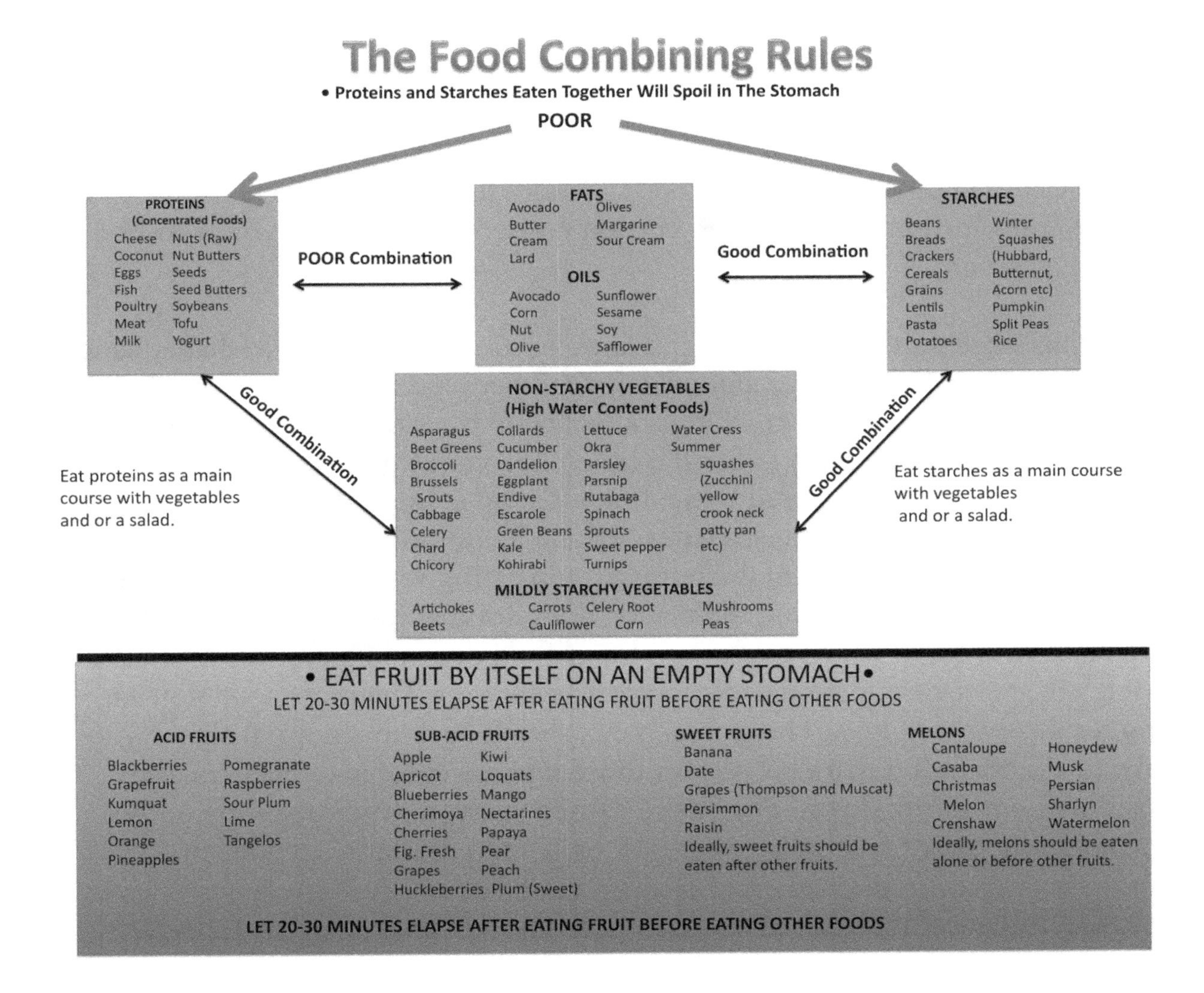


**Food chart adapted from NSP Products.

# Daryl's How to Eat Guide

**Eat five to six small meals per day**

The stomach is a little bit bigger than your fist. This is why we need to eat small amounts of food per feeding. If we were supposed to eat large quantities the stomach would be very large. The stomach is small and is designed to hold small amounts of food. In order to keep your digestive system working effectively it is important to eat small meals throughout the day. Five to six small meals per day is ideal. Eating like this will keep your VNES working efficiently, will cause a boosting effect to the metabolism and will actually raise the temperature of the digestive system thus increasing fat metabolism. However, you must eat highly dense nutrient foods to have this effect occur. Eating junk food will produce ill results. The more nutrient-dense the food the more the intestines have to work to breakdown the nutrients. Also, when you eat nutrient-dense foods you won't be able to eat as much.

Avoid eating large portions. I consider a large portion anything more than a hand size. If you constantly eat large amounts of food per feeding you will stretch your stomach and intestines. There are nerves attached to the stomach that signal the brain to eat. Once the stomach is full the lining becomes tight. This tautness causes the nerves to send a signal to the brain to stop eating. If you chronically overeat then the stomach lining stretches beyond its normal limit. The nerve receptors that turn on and signal the brain to stop eating won't respond until the stomach is fully taut. As a result, the person does not feel full and continues to fill the stomach with food, which could be a lot of food depending on how much the stomach has to stretch for the nerve receptors to turn on. The more food you eat, the bigger the stomach gets. The stomach can shrink back to a normal size if you eat five to six meals a day. However, for those that are chronic overeaters, the stomach will not shrink down. They have caused such an over stretching of the stomach that the nerve receptors never turn on to stop the eating sequence.

Here is the sequence of steps the stomach goes through during an eating cycle:
1. The stomach empties. The nerve receptors signal the brain to start eating.
2. Food is delivered and the stomach is filled causing the lining to become taut.
3. Nerve receptors signal the brain to stop eating.

The idea is to keep the stomach small by eating small, nutrient-dense foods. Avoid overeating!

**Control your eating -- slow down**

Eating food should be a controlled, methodical process. We live in a highly competitive, fast-paced society. Everything is based on how quickly can we get things done so that we can do more. This Type-A behavior usually causes people to eat faster. When you engulf food, too much air is consumed, causing poor digestion. When putting food into the mouth it is important to chew it completely. There are digestive enzymes in the saliva that help break down the food. Food is a foreign substance until it mixes with our own digestive enzymes. Once the food is fully mixed it then enters the stomach where the more potent digestive enzymes do their work. The more you can chew in the mouth the less work the stomach has to do to breakdown the food. Thorough chewing also prevents the accumulation of air, reducing the bloating and gas often associated with indigestion. Chew your food completely. Slow down and do not rush the process.

**Get control of your emotions**

Too much stress hypes up the sympathetic nervous system and can cause a release of cortisol, inhibiting protein synthesis and fat burning.

**No Smoking**

Smoking restricts the capillaries, preventing, oxygen to enter cells and disrupts normal muscle metabolism, reduces muscle cell size, destroys Vitamin B and C uptake in the blood, and increases free radial production.

**Eat only one to two different types of food at a time**

The body is designed to only digest one type of food at a time. When you put too many foods into the mix you develop digestive distress (as discussed earlier). The less the body has to sort out many different foods the faster the nutrients get into the body. Eating only a couple of foods at a time will also help determine if you are allergic to a certain food. If you are allergic then you can simply identify to the food and eliminate it. Food allergies are not as easy to identify when you eat many foods altogether.

**It's how much you digest that counts, not calories**

So many people are fixated on thinking about calories. It is not about calories, it is about how many nutrients you digest. Proper digestion is crucial for good health. Chronic poor digestion can lead to many health problems. The disease known as acid reflux is not a disease at all. Acid reflux is a result of poor digestion where hydrochloric acid builds up in the stomach and is forced up into the esophagus. Build up of food gets stuck in the intestines and is unable to break down. Digestive acid cannot penetrate, and it forms a regurgitating effect. The intestines are comprised of yeast, parasites and bacteria. There are both good and bad forms of yeast, parasites and bacteria in the intestines. Poor digestion will promote more bad forms of parasites, bacteria, and fungi and increase the formation of yeast. This increase in pathogens will begin to weaken the nutrient supply being delivered into the blood, thus increasing the aging effect and producing illness.

Poor digestion can also lead to the insufficient breakdown of essential fatty acids. Essential fatty acids are important for many functions of the body. If you do not get enough essential fatty acids into you diet, then the blood system becomes compromised. Essential fatty acids are fats that the body cannot manufacture. You must get essential fatty acids from good healthy food sources.

**Digestive enzyme support**

The more you break down the food before it enters the small intestines, the greater the nutrient absorption. Taking a digestive enzyme supplement with each meal can help aid the breakdown process in the stomach and intestines. Digestive enzymes are safe and have no side effects. They are simply an aid that provides additional enzymatic support to breakdown food. You can find digestive enzymes in any natural food store. Hydrochloric acid is important for the breakdown of nutrients. The intestines need to have a high acid base medium for proper digestion to occur. Acidity helps defend against the development of yeast, parasites, mutations, viruses, and bacteria.

**Always eat some protein before retiring for the night**

While you sleep the body goes into a fasting mode. It is beneficial to have some protein in the digestive tract during this time. Proteins release growth factors that help repair cells. The body only grows during the sleep cycle. Going to bed on an empty stomach can cause the body to go into a catabolic state using its own internal protein to repair damaged cells, which is not desirable.

**Always eat protein upon rising**

Night sleep is a fasting process. During sleep the body recovers from daily cellular damage. Normal sleep patterns will create a balance in homeostatic processes. By the time a person wakes up he/she should feel refreshed and energized. There should be no need for sugar when you awaken. Sugar metabolism is regulated during the sleeping cycle and should not be a factor when you wake up. It is important not to force the sympathetic system to fire up first thing in the morning. The sympathetic nervous system is fueled by sugar. Once you consume sugar and set off the insulin response, fatigue usually sets in shortly after. If you set off this sequence the first thing in the morning, you are at a disadvantage for the rest of the day. Chances are you will continue to eat sugary foods to keep your energy up. Overeating sugar will provide a false serotonin boost. Serotonin is a monoamine neurotransmitter that helps regulate mood, appetite, sleep, muscular contractions, and memory. During normal cycles of brain activity, serotonin, provides a boost in mood. When serotonin levels drop the central nervous system becomes depressed. The brain perceives that the blood sugar is elevated and activates the sequence of hormones to boost the central nervous system. This reaction is only short lived. Once the pancreas realizes that there is too much sugar in the bloodstream it releases insulin from the islets of langerhans cells. Insulin clears out the sugar from the bloodstream. When blood sugar levels drop, the excitatory hormones are then turned off, depressing the central nervous system (CNS). In order to boost the CNS, sugar must be present to activate the excitatory hormonal sequence again.

People who are addicted to eating carbohydrates are constantly forcing their sympathetic nervous system to turn on. This releases excitatory hormones and results in an acute boost of energy. To avoid the peaks and valleys of loading the body with sugar throughout the day, it is important to start the day with a protein.

Eating protein helps maintain blood-sugar levels. Insulin is not released when protein enters the bloodstream. Also, eating protein will break the fasting cycle that is associated with sleeping. Breakfast simply means *break the fasting.* The first thing you eat when you wake up will set the precedence for the rest of the day. You can eat low glycemic complex carbohydrates in the morning, but eat them a couple hours after ingesting protein. This will provide slow burning sugar to fuel your blood for the remainder of the day. However, the first thing you should eat upon waking is a protein. As I discussed earlier, protein only last three hours in the bloodstream after digestion. It is important to get it into your body as soon as you wake up to give it time to digest and be utilized in the bloodstream. By not eating protein first thing in the morning you could be at risk of developing sugar cravings throughout the day.

Personally, I have noticed a dramatic difference in the appearance of my body if I don't eat enough protein throughout the day. As an experiment I ate only carbs for three days. The results were: I was tired all the time, moody, my muscle measurements decreased, I lost strength and I craved sugar. As soon as I incorporated protein back into my meal plan I instantly felt a difference. My strength came back, my muscles felt full and hard, my energy was high, and I didn't crave sugars. I am convinced that protein is the most important nutrient to consume first thing in the morning.

**Eat fat with protein**

It is important to eat fat with protein. Eating egg whites without the yolk will only produce sugar in the bloodstream. This is because fat has to accompany protein to allow the protein to hydrolyze through the liver. Without fat the protein will be broken down into sugar. Always eat a fat with a protein. Most meats, eggs, and cheese contain fat and protein in the correct ratios. Separating fat from these foods changes the metabolic ratios.

**Avoid drinking coffee**

It is an American ritual to wake up and drink a cup of coffee to wake up. I find this to be counterproductive. If you need to drink a stimulant to wake you up then you must figure out what is making you tired in the first place. When you wake up you should be completely refreshed and energized. If you are not energized then you have to look at a few variables to determine why you are sluggish:

- Did you eat carbohydrates before going to bed?
- Did you have a rough night of sleep (insomnia)?
- Are you suffering from depression?
- Are you overtraining?
- Are you malnourished?

In humans, caffeine is a central nervous system stimulant. Caffeine produces an alert state in the body and helps ward off drowsiness. Too much caffeine can have an adverse effect on cortisol production and the adrenal gland function. Cortisol is an inhibitory hormone that shuts off the permeability of cells during times of stress. When cortisol is released in the blood, fat metabolism ceases. Another effect from consuming too much caffeine is adrenal exhaustion. I believe that drinking 3-6 cups of coffee per day activates the sympathetic nervous system to the point of adrenal exhaustion. Adrenal glands are designed to release: cortisol, adrenaline, corticosteroids and catecholamines during times of sympathetic nervous system activation. Small amounts of stress hormone secretion from the adrenal glands are normal and produce few side effects. Over production of stress hormones secreted by the adrenal glands can cause the adrenals to burn out; this is known as *adrenal exhaustion.*

Adrenal exhaustion can result in excessive fatigue and physical exhaustion, non-refreshing sleep, overwhelmed feelings, salt and sugar cravings, difficulty concentrating, poor digestion, low immune functioning, food or environmental allergies, chronic low blood pressure, extreme sensitivity to cold, insomnia, poor exercise recovery, an ability to recover from illness, and an increase in abdominal fat.

**Do not over drink fluids with food (water, juices, alcohol, soda, milk)**
In order for proper digestion, hydrochloric (HCL) acid needs to be in complete concentration. Drinking too much liquid with food will dilute HCL making digestion difficult. Protein digestion can be hindered if HCL levels are low. The bile that is used to help digest protein becomes ineffective. Bile will float to the top of diluted HCL. Burping, having severe gas, bloating, diarrhea, nausea, weakness, sweating, increased blood pressure, and headaches are all symptoms of poor digestion and diluted HCL concentrations. Mixing too much fluid with food will result in poor digestion.

**Take a tablespoon of apple cider vinegar**
If you have a tough time digesting food try taking a tablespoon of apple cider vinegar before eating. This will help enhance the digestive properties to better assist in the breakdown of food. Also, if you are going to be eating starchy foods, taking a tablespoon of cider vinegar before eating will help neutralize the sugar in the intestines, reducing an insulin reaction. The best kind of apple cider vinegar is Braggs. Braggs is a real source of organic apple cider vinegar.

**Rest after you eat**
We live in a fast paced world. We eat fast foods because we don't have time to eat. We take stimulants to keep us awake. We crave instant gratification. This fast paced lifestyle wreaks havoc on the digestive system. Fast eating constricts the intestines, making it hard for food to digest completely. Sit back with your feet up and relax for a about 10-20 minutes after eating to allow for proper digestion.

**Sodium bicarbonate**
Ingesting a small amount of sodium bicarbonate (pill form) before exercise has been known to help prolong the aerobic and anaerobic systems of the muscle. Sodium bicarbonate is an alkalizing agent that buffers acid out of the blood stream. Sodium bicarbonate cannot permeate into a muscle cell. However, the excess acid that leaks out of the muscle cell interacts with the sodium bicarbonate and is buffered. This allows the blood acidic level to stay low for longer periods reducing long term fatigue factors, thus allowing the aerobic and anaerobic systems of the muscles to work more effectively.

Sodium bicarbonate has also been known to reduce fungi in the body. Fungus (candida and yeast) is in everybody. If the levels of fungi increase beyond a normal level then disease can develop. Cancer has been considered in the category of a fungus. Consuming a small amount of sodium bicarbonate periodically can help remove certain fungi in the bloodstream. I am not suggesting that sodium bicarbonate is a cure for cancer, but there is no evidence to support that it can not help prevent it.

**Raw Honey**
Raw honey has been around for centuries and has many benefits. Honey was once considered a power food in biblical times. It was believed that Sampson ate raw honey for his strength. Raw honey aides in digestion. The inverted sugar is easily assimilated through the intestines, reducing the risk of bacterial radicals from developing. The fatty acids help stimulate the peristalsis of the intestines. Raw honey is complete in carbohydrates, amino acids, vitamins, minerals, enzymes and phytonutrients, plus helps strengthen the immune system. I recommend taking a tablespoon a day. If you develop a sore throat, have some natural honey and it can help soothe the irritated area, and the enzymes help attack the bacteria. For a boost in your workout, ingest a tablespoon thirty minutes before exercising.

**Celtic Sea Salt**
Celtic sea salt is a healthy alternative to table salt. It helps with balancing the body's alkaline and acid levels. It helps restore good digestion and increases energy. Sea salt supplies all eighty-two trace minerals the body needs to help support cellular production. There is naturally occurring iodine that helps against radiation and other pollutants. Sea salt has been known to help reduce allergic reactions to airborne irritants. Sea salt should be incorporated in a healthy nutrition plan on a daily basis. All you need is a teaspoon per day.

**Garlic**
Garlic has been around for centuries and it provides the following:
- It is a natural antibiotic
- It prevents common colds
- It can help treat some forms of acne
- Garlic has blood cleansing properties. It can help reduce the low density lipoproteins (LDL cholesterol) in the blood
- It has blood clotting factors; be careful of taking garlic if you are on anticoagulants
- Ward off vampires ( just kidding, I couldn't resist)

Garlic is most effective when eaten raw. Chopped and crushed is best.
If you don't want the bad breath associated with eating garlic you can take an odorless garlic supplement instead.

# Supplements

In today's world, I feel that it is essential to take supplements. Supplements are powerful foods, vitamins and minerals that help supply the body with vital nutrients that we cannot get from food alone. Unfortunately, finding healthy nutrients in the foods that we eat is becoming more difficult these days. Processing and the manipulation of natural foods, along with the natural depletion of vital minerals from the earth is reason enough to add supplements to your daily meal schedule. Here are the supplements I suggest that everyone take on a daily basis.

***** Please note: If you have any type of medical condition or are not sure how supplements will react in your system, I recommend consulting a natural nutritionist or a homeopathic doctor before taking any supplement.***

***<u>The following are the supplements I recommend for optimal health.</u> However, in Appendix II there is a list of many of the modern day supplements that are used for health, weight loss, endurance, mental acuity, and sleep. I suggest that you gather as much information about a particular supplement before taking it. Supplements react differently to each person's bio-individuality. Never take supplements without prior knowledge of their effectiveness.***

**Olive Leaf**
Is a great virus and bacteria killer. It also keeps latent viruses from emerging. Olive leaf is an ancient herbal medicine that helps fight against sickness and disease. Take one to two tablets per day.

**Alfalfa**
Alfalfa (father of all foods) is a powerful food that has been known for lowering cholesterol levels, aiding in digestion, defending against peptic ulcers; it is a great diuretic and bowel regulator, and helps kidney function. This is an overlooked supplement that is loaded with benefits. It has a very high protein ratio containing all eight essential amino acids, vitamins and minerals, and calcium. Calcium is an important mineral for the contractions of muscle tissue.

Contains eight essential enzymes:
1. Lipase - helps fat metabolism
2. Amylase- metabolizes starch
3. Coagulase - forms blood clot factors
4. Emulsin- breaks down sugar.

5. Invertase- sugar metabolism.
6. Peroxidate- blood oxidizer
7. Pectinase- forms vegetable jelly.
8. Protase- helps metabolize protein.

Take 4-8 tablets per day.

**Glandulars (Sterol 11)**
"Like glands nourish like glands." Glandulars are extracted from animal glands. Animal glands are loaded with protein, essential fat, vitamins and minerals. Raw glandulars, when entered into the body, attract to like glands, i.e, kidney feeds kidney, brain feeds brain, etcetera.

**Wheat Germ Oil***:* is a great hormone precursor that helps fight free radicals and tissue repair. It is best taken on an empty stomach following workouts.

**Kelp:** Contains 44 minerals, and has a high iodine ratio. Helps activate the production of the thyroid gland. People who suffer from low thyroid activity can take kelp to help re-establish natural thyroid production.

**Dessicatted Liver:** This is another overlooked supplement. Dessicatted liver has a high protein ratio that is absorbed in the body without having to go through liver hydrolysis. It supports the building of blood. It is a good anti-catabolic food that helps boost testosterone levels.

Here is an excerpt by my friend Ron Kosloff about dessicatted liver:
*Only within the past few years have the important values of Beef Liver Extract been proven and new light shed on this outstanding food. One of the most important facts about Beef Liver Extract is its ability to detoxify many chemicals hazardous to the body and very difficult to avoid. Most of the meats we eat contain the dangerous hormone D.E.S. With sufficient daily intake of Beef Liver Extract, the body can detoxify cortisone, nicotine, alcohol, marijuana, and many pharmaceutical drugs. Only recently has the most important fact about Beef Liver Extract been discovered-the presence of P-450. P-450 is a catalyst which speeds up the oxidation of chemicals important to human life and detoxifies the poisonous substances we breathe in and ingest. Production of energy is a process of oxidation of glucose within the body. This in turn produces "fatigue" toxins that gradually slow down energy. P-450 can improve the energy production process and improve the body's ability to detoxify the "fatigue" toxins.*

*P-450 is not water soluble, and the vacuum drying process does not remove this newly discovered liver factor, instead it concentrates it.*

*It took Dr. Minor P. Coon of the University of Michigan 20 years to isolate the red protein pigment, named P-450. The extensive laboratory testing proved that P-450 was able to perform all the functions of liver that had been previously tested on vitamins but not found attributed to them. Later tests on children were performed. The results were confirmed. The P-450 found in liver extract is important to human growth.*

**Digestive Enzymes:** In order to properly digest food it is essential that there is a good concentration of digestive enzymes in the stomach and intestines. Hydrocholoric acid is a key component in the stomach and intestines for breaking down food. If food is not broken down adequately enough, nutrient absorption is compromised. By taking 1-2 digestive enzymes before you eat will ensure the proper breakdown of protein, fats, and carbohydrates.

**Amino Acids:** Amino acids are the building blocks of protein, and therefore are the foundation for building muscle. There are two types of amino acids: *essential* and *non-essential.* Essential amino acids are not synthesized in the body must be derived from food. There are nine essential amino acids. Non-essential aminos are the twelve amino acids that are synthesized by the body. Supplementing with essential amino acids has been very successful in adults and is considered one of the basics of all supplement programs.

There are two types of amino supplements that are important, *free form* and *branch chained.* ***Free form amino acids*** are a collection of all nine essential amino acids that can be taken at any time. ***Branched chain amino acids*** only consist of three amino acids that are bound to each other: L-leucine, L-isoleucine, and L-valine. L-Leucine is considered a vital anabolic amino acid that plays a major role in the maintenance and building of muscle. Too little L-leucine can spell disaster to muscle and put the body into a catabolic state. L-Leucine also helps in the production the energy. Taking branched chain amino acids throughout the day and before going to bed is recommended for maximum results.

The great thing about taking amino acids (free form and branched chain), is that they are safe, and have no side effects. They both bypass being hydrolyzed in the liver and go directly in the bloodstream. Less stress for the liver to contend with and less work for the kidneys make amino acid supplements a great foundation to building muscle.

**Mineral Complex**
Minerals are essential for proper cellular function. The Earth's mineral supply is decreasing. It is important to take a mineral supplement to ensure that you get the required amount of minerals per day to feed the VNES.

**Vitamin Packs**
The foundation of a nutrition program. A time-released vitamin and mineral pack taken daily is a great way to provide the body with required nutrients. Time released vitamins have a certain time that that they stay active in the system. Time released vitamins stay in the small intestines and flake off, binding with food as it passes through into the portal vein.

**I/KI Thyroid Support**
For thyroid health. Iodine is the most essential nutrient for the function of your thyroid. This is an important supplement to take for both men and women.

**Power Food:** These are food wafers loaded with vitamins, minerals, and glandulars that supply the body the necessary amount of nutrients per serving. These wafers can be used as a snack in between meals or used for a meal replacement. This product is a great addition to any meal plan.

**Raw Revolution Food Organic Live Food Bar:** These bars follow my raw food philosophy and they taste great. I highly recommend these bars as a snack. www.rawrev.com

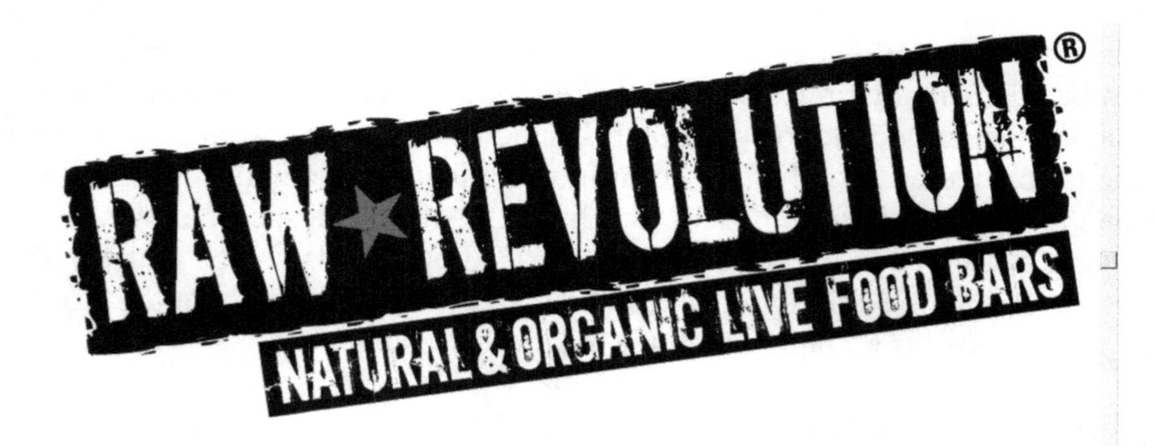

# Raw Food: Nature's Way

Earth is a mysterious world. Its origin and purpose are not known. What we do know is that Earth is a living, breathing entity. At one time the Earth was rich in nutrients and organic compounds. Now the Earth is running out of its natural resources. The surface of the Earth is losing its mineral levels. Food is being depleted of its vitamins and animal proteins are being subjected to environmental poisons. Ever since the beginning of the industrial age, pollutants have infiltrated into the Earths atmosphere. For over the past hundred years toxic waste has been emitted into the air. Acid raid is a result of toxic pollution. Acid rain falls down on the Earth and destroys crops, vegetation, and air quality. Animals then eat the grass that has been affected by acid rain. We eat animals, therefore we take in the by-products of toxic rain. This cycle of toxic ecology is what will eventually destroy our natural resources for good.

A hundred years ago it was rare to hear of someone dying of breast cancer, colon cancer, melanoma, pancreatic cancer, or prostate cancer. Though these diseases existed, they contributed to less than one quarter of the mortality rate at that time. Now a hundred years later, it is estimated that one out of every three Americans will develop one of these conditions in their lifetime. I believe that the reason for many of the diseases that affect Americans today is toxic ecology. The days of organic, natural raw food are dying out.

Farms were once the staple of the American way of life. There were no pesticides, preservatives or other pollutants to destroy the natural food products. Now it is rare to find a working farm that uses no chemicals on the crops. If you search hard enough you might find an organic farm that doesn't use pesticides or harmful chemicals on their crops, but this is rare. This is a shame.

Sticking to raw organic foods is the best for the body. However, even though a food is labeled as organic does not mean that all organic foods are truly safe from toxins. However, they have far less chemicals in them than non-organic foods do. Raw food contains active enzymes that are not damaged from processing or cooking procedures. Cooking raw vegetables changes the molecular chains of the food and kills live active enzymes making the food less valuable. Raw foods are straight from the natural matrix of the Earth. I suggest eating raw foods as the staple of your nutritional plan.

### Cooking Food

Raw foods contain all the vital enzymes and nutrients necessary for feeding the cells of the body. When food is cooked the nutrients are destroyed. Here are my suggestions for cooking food.

- **Never use a microwave** to cook food. Microwave ovens emit radiation and mutate the molecular structure of the food, making the food valueless and cancer producing.

- **Don't fry food in fat** Fryolators heat up saturated fat and break down the hydrogen bonds producing trans fatty acids. Trans-fatty acids are unhealthy fats that contribute to cardiovascular disease. Fried food should be avoided. Also, Vitamin B1 and Pantothenic acid are destroyed in meat from frying.

- **Never over cook vegetables** The minute a vegetable is picked from its stem the nutrient value diminishes quite rapidly. By the time you purchase the vegetable and bring it home, more nutrients have been lost. Now, if you cook it you will lose even more of the nutrient value. If you overcook it you have pretty much wiped out all the nutrients, making the vegetable worthless. Boiling vegetables in water is not a good idea either because the hot water leaches out the nutrients from the food. Steaming is the best method for cooking vegetables.

- **Broil or bake your meat** Salmonella is a bacteria that causes infectious disease in humans. Eating raw meats is not advised for this reason. However, most salmonella bacteria lives on the outside layer of the meat. So, if you cook the outside of the meat it reduces the risk of ingesting salmonella bacteria. E Coli is another bacteria that causes illness. E Coli is usually found in beef and/or spinach. E Coli, in meat, is often attributed to fecal matter from the animal being on the outside of the meat. This causes a growth of E Coli, which is dangerous. However, cooking the outside layers of the meat you can reduce the risk of E Coli. It is important to retain as much of the essential enzymes of the protein by keeping the center of the meat pink or bloody. The more you cook the meat the more you destroy the protein. Be careful not to overcook the meat or to blacken the outside layers, doing so will damage the fat.

- **Avoid cooking with polyunsaturated fats** The high heat damages the molecular structure of the fat making it undigestible. The best fats to cook with are saturated and monounsaturated fats (refer to the fat section).

- **Crock pot cooking can cause nutrient depletion** Vegetables left in a crock pot all day will lose vital nutrients. Also, the fat will be absorbed from the meat. It is best to lightly steam the vegetables and add them to the crock pot for 5-10 minutes to create flavor before serving.

- **Steaming** is a better choice for cooking vegetables and fruits. The heat is moist and only takes a few minutes to cook the vegetable, so less nutrients are lost.

- **Avoid drinking fruit juices from concentrate**. The concentration process extracts water out of the fruit leaving only the sugar available. The sugar is then diluted with water to make more product. This allows companies to spread out the content of the fruit making more money. The concentration process breaks down the original molecular structure of the fruit making it a high glycemic substance. In fact, with the exception of unsweetened fruit juices for fasting programs, I would not recommend drinking juices at all. Orange juice is thought to be a good source of Vitamin C, but is also has a high glycemic index that activates the insulin sequence.

- **Food should be refrigerated** as soon as possible. Vitamins and minerals will retain their value better. Eating the freshest food reduces nutrient depletion.

Sometimes I feel like I live separately from the rest of the world when it comes to nutrition. When I started learning about nutrition I was in college. The college classes focused on the FDA (Food and Drug Administration) guidelines. The more I studied the material the more I disagreed with it. Then I came across two men who helped pave my way into a whole new realm of nutrition consciousness, Ron Kosloff and Vince Gironda. What I learned from these two men gave me the direction I needed to broaden my own basic knowledge of nutrition.

There must be more to life than we know. I don't believe that we as human beings have truly tapped into the power this Earth has to provide. We are all subjected to the garbage that the food industry has to serve. No one seems to be fighting against all the destruction that food companies are doing to our natural food sources. I am angry to constantly see and hear all the commercials about junk foods. This country is deplorable when it comes to nutrition. To think that if you eat what the FDA approves as healthy, you will end up getting sick or developing disease from it. There is something wrong with this system. The culprits of the declining health in America are the big food corporations and the FDA. The FDA doesn't regulate the harmful chemicals that are being pumped into the foods that are readily available to everyone in America. Every second on television there is a commercial selling some form of junk food, brainwashing us into thinking that it is good for us. I am a bit annoyed at the lack of the governmental industry's defense of our health. Most of the problems associated with our health care are directly linked to the poisons that are in our foods, which can be found right in your friendly neighborhood grocery store.

I wonder if the government really cares about trying to keep people healthy, or are they concerned with polluting our systems so that we have to purchase drugs to control our illness symptoms. I can't believe that we live in a world where you can get seriously ill from eating food produced by food companies. The evolution of nutrition is not progressing toward the betterment of mankind. In fact, it is just the opposite. Earthly nutrition intelligence is infantile in development. We have not even come close to what our true purpose here on earth is. Human beings have gotten away from what they really are--cells made up of atoms and molecules. We are all a part of a universal energy that cannot be separated. Present day human beings have lost the connection between their true identity and the earth. People are plugged into technology and have lost touch with universal reality.

The foundation of our existence is based on healthy nutrients. Without healthy nutrients we become ill, or worse, die. I don't think that we were meant to live by the support of medications. I feel that many diseases can be resolved with proper nutrition. However, it is hard to find real nutrients anymore. It is a bit scary to think about the possibility that organic farms will one day be shut down and food companies will totally control everything we eat. If this ever happens, then we are all in trouble because live nutrients will be replaced by artificial byproducts and toxic chemicals that serve no purpose in the human body. This is already happening. The more processed food you eat, the greater the chance you have of getting ill or developing disease.

I am upset that not more people are fighting for the right to produce real organic foods in this country. The Earth provides us with the means to live, but we are destroying it. If we continue to deplete the Earth's natural resources of nutrients the human species will not survive. Life will not be sustainable.

What we can do to reverse this trend is to learn as much as possible about nutrition to help create some type of positive awareness. When I see overweight people, or people that are suffering from ailments related to malnutrition it upsets me. I am not upset with those affected, I am upset with the companies that produce the foods that cause this to happen. I know that some people don't have the means to purchase the "good food" and have to resort to purchasing low nutrient, chemically ladened foods. It should never even have to come to this. I believe that we all should be able to afford eating healthy organic foods. To think that only wealthier people are the ones that can afford the best sources of food and receive the best health care, while the less fortunate have to settle for cheaper, poisoned food and an inadequate health care system is depressing. There is something seriously wrong with this situation.

We live in an unconscious world that lives in the darkness of our reality. There is a light that is trying to shine through the darkness, but we refuse to see it. Perhaps someday the light will shine and the people will understand their true reality. Unfortunately, this probably will never happen.

We are all connected into the living matrix of this universe. Life on Earth is based on a give-and-take relationship. We give carbon dioxide to the Earth's atmosphere by expiring air from our lungs, and in return the Earth provides us with oxygen from the trees. Without either one of these gases life on earth would not be possible. If we continue to destroy the Earth's surface (trees and vegetation) the gas exchange system could be compromised. An imbalance in the natural gases of the Earths atmosphere can directly hinder the development of natural food sources. When natural food sources are compromised so is our health. Human beings are connected to the Earth and depend on its natural resources for survival. Once the Earth's natural resources are depleted then life as we know it may no longer exist.

If you pretend to ascend into space and look back at the Earth as a whole then you could understand what I am talking about. When you are in space looking at Earth you can't see the people or the buildings etcetera. You only see the global sphere of Earth. Now, if I was a scientist looking at Earth through a microscope I would see a cell that was dying. What I would see is a high level of active cells (animals, humans) trying to defend against the antibody invaders. You would notice fluctuations in temperatures. You would notice that the cells on earth were diseased and dying out at a fast rate. You would notice the water supply, the vitamin and mineral supply, and the overall nutrient chain being critically depleted.

This world could be such a great resource of health. But due to a regressed social unconsciousness, we will never see a change. In fact, it will only get worse. The ignorance of man will destroy mankind. Perhaps the Earth will have enough of our foolishness and destroy its outer layer, thus destroying all of civilization in order to cleanse itself and restart another life system!

Since I cannot change the world and create total social consciousness, I can only provide my interpretation on how humans should eat. Perhaps one day there will be a shift in social consciousness forcing people to wake up from their unconscious sleep and become more aware of the need for good nutrition on this planet.

**Eat raw foods whenever possible**

Food holds within itself the basis of life. Nutrients are sensitive to so many factors so they need to be treated with care. Many foods are damaged through all the processing methods. Our bodies are in a raw state and we need to eat raw foods to feed the cells. Cooking and the processing of food kills vital nutrients. I believe that all food, with the exception of meats, should be eaten in their raw state so the enzymes and nutrients are actively ingested and absorbed. The earth provides food for us to eat. Fruit and vegetables are not meant to be cooked. Yet, everyone is always cooking them. The only exception to cooking fruits would be for someone who suffers from an intestinal disease such as Crohn's disease. In this case steaming fruit is permissible. Steaming softens the skin and helps break down the fiber, making it easier for the intestines to digest.

The beginning to a healthy body is to consume raw natural foods. Raw foods are any kind of food that is complete within itself. For example, vegetables, fruits, and sushi. Cooking and processing destroy the natural elements of food. There are certain foods that should be cooked to prevent getting a food-borne illness. Eggs can be eaten raw but many people feel that this is not healthy. If you feel the need to cook eggs, then you should lightly scramble them. Never over cook eggs, as this destroys the fat and protein content. Hard boiled eggs are not good. Once the egg gets hard, the quality of the protein and fat are reduced significantly.

Never eat just the egg whites without eating the yolk. Many people are afraid of eating egg yolks. They have been told that they will die from a heart attack if they habitually eat egg yolks. This is ridiculous! If you throw away the egg yolk and just eat the white the liver will convert the protein into sugar. You might think that you are doing a healthy thing by throwing out the yolk, which contains the good cholesterol that the body needs, but in actuality you are converting the protein into sugar. If you continue to eat low-fat foods you will run the risk of developing high cholesterol. Protein must be accompanied by essential fat to hydrolyze through the liver.

**Limit protein intake per meal**

The recommended protein allowance per meal is thirty grams. Eating too much protein will store as fat, be converted into sugar, or be eliminated in the urine. Do not ingest protein too fast. Take time to chew your food completely. Doing this allows the digestive enzymes to do a better job of breaking the food down into smaller constituents.

**Eat small meals throughout the day**

The stomach is small and doesn't need to be over-filled. Forcing large amounts of food into the stomach will cause it to stretch to an undesirable size, making digestion more difficult. The best method to employ is to eat small meals. This will promote less stress for the digestive system and allow for better nutrient exchange. Each meal should consist of the right combination of food.

**A Correct Food Table To Follow**

When I was in school I learned the silly food pyramid chart. This chart was developed to provide Americans with the correct number of servings of each food we should consume on a daily basis. It suggests that we should all eat 2-3 servings of protein a day, 5-6 fruits and vegetables a day, and 10-12 servings of carbohydrates per day. This food pyramid promotes only one goal -- OBESITY. Because any American who eats 10-12 servings of carbohydrates a day will surely become over fat or obese.

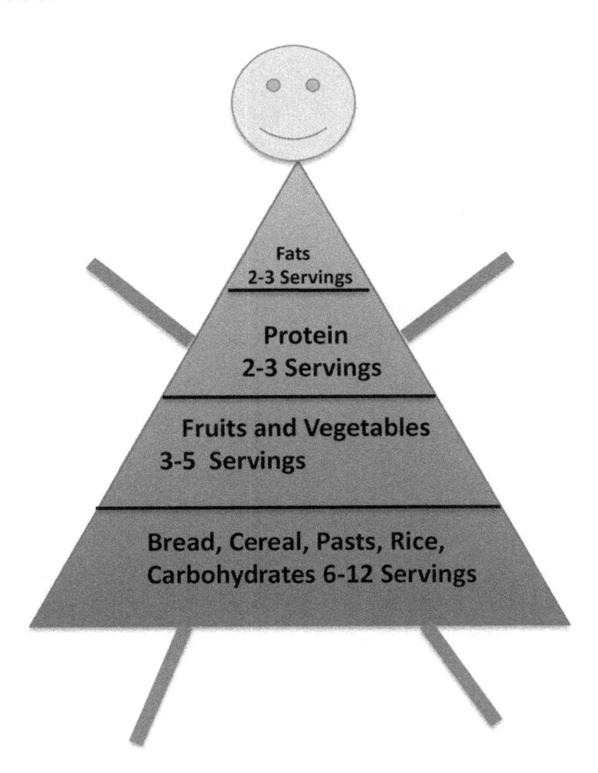


You end up looking like the pyramid if you eat according to it!

To make it easier for you to make better choices in your nutrition plan, I have made some changes to the food pyramid. In fact, I have made it into a square with four equal parts. I call it **Conant's Dietary Food Chart**.

How it works is simple. Try to consume foods more toward the center of the square. The foods on the outskirts should be AVOIDED. Unfortunately, many Americans live on the outskirts of the square. Poor choices will result in poor health. There are thousands of foods out there and too many to write down, so I decided to put the most popular foods consumed by people in the square. Earth foods are the best. Earth foods are natural foods that come from the Earth. Once the Earth food gets stripped of its nutrients through processing or are tampered with, the value of the food drops. The food is then put into the poor choice category. The more man has tampered with the food the less value it has.

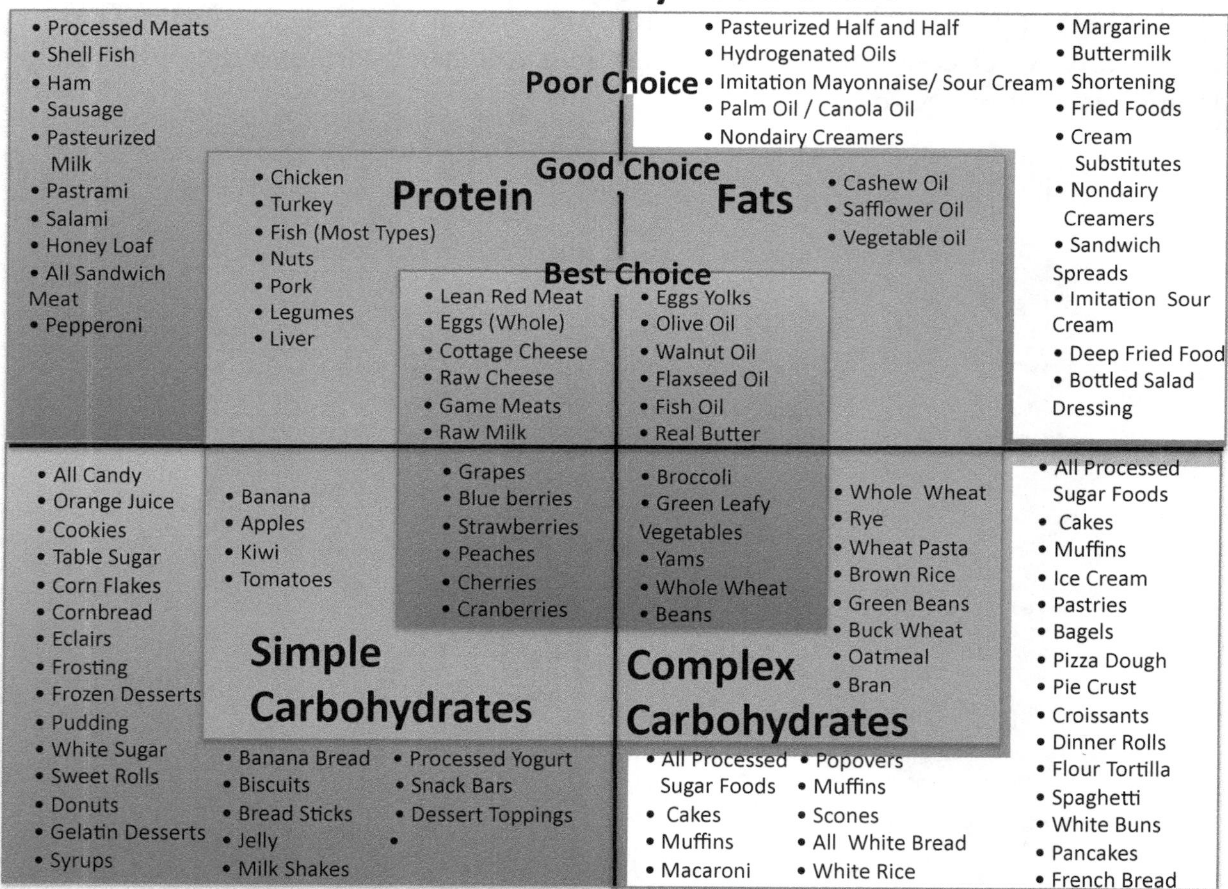

Stay within the center of the square for the best nutrition. Keep food in its natural state, raw (as much as possible, exception with meats), unprocessed, and chemical free.

Once you understand the food square, you can use it as a quick guide to determine the value of the food you are about to eat.

The following is the daily vital nutrient requirement intake chart. This is how much protein, carbs, and fats you should consume daily. Consuming the best food sources helps promote greater health and vitality.

Here are the steps to take before eating any type of food.

1. First, look at the nutrient value of the food (fats, proteins, carbs, etc.). Does it provide the best source of nutrients?
2. Can it be eaten in its raw state? Is it processed by man?
3. Does it fall into the right combination for proper digestion?
4. Is the entire meal the size of your hand?
5. Does the sugar content fall into the safe category or does it alert the sugar radar?

## Vital Nutrient Exchange

*The Basis Of Cellular Life*

| | | DIETARY INTAKE |
|---|---|---|
| DAILY VITAL NUTRIENT REQUIREMENT | Macro **Protein** Micro | ***High Quality:*** 5-6 Servings Per Day.<br>***Uptake Time:*** 2-3 Hours<br>***Blood Stream Life:*** 2-3 Hours<br>***MUST BE REPLENISHED FREQUENTLY*** |
| | Macro **Carbs** Micro | ***Low Glycemic:*** 5-6 Servings Per Day.<br>***Uptake Time:*** 30m-1Hour<br>***Blood Stream Life:*** 2-3 Hours<br>***AVOID HIGH GLYCEMIC FOODS*** |
| | Macro **Fats** Micro | ***Natural Fats:*** 5-6 Servings Per Day.<br>***Uptake Time:*** 2-3Hour<br>***Blood Stream Life:*** 4-6 Hours<br>***AVOID TRANS FATTY ACIDS*** |
| | Vits / Minerals | ***Found in a variety of healthy nutrient Dense foods. Supplement if necessary.*** |

By following these simple steps you can always be on the right track with your nutrition. It does not get any easier than this, folks!

## Vital Nutrient Exchange

*The Basis Of Cellular Life*

| DAILY VITAL NUTRIENT REQUIREMENT | | Good Sources | Poor Sources |
|---|---|---|---|
| | Macro Protein Micro | • Lean Meats<br>• Eggs<br>• Cheese<br>• Nuts | • Processed Meat<br>• Man Made<br>• Nitrate Ridden<br>• Chemical Ridden<br>• Preservatives |
| | Macro Carbs Micro | • Green Leafy Vegetables<br>• Multi-Grains<br>• Fruit with Skin | • Simple Sugars<br>• Pasta (white)<br>• Sugary Drinks<br>• Enriched Foods<br>• Man Made |
| | Macro Fats Micro | • Lean Meats<br>• Eggs<br>• Cheese<br>• Nuts | • Processed Meat<br>• Man Made<br>• Trans Fatty Acid<br>• Chemical Ridden<br>• Hydrolysized |
| | Vits / Minerals | • A variety of Good Foods | • All Junk Foods<br>• Enriched Foods |

## We All Must Take Inventory of Ourselves

The intent of this book was not to provide you with tons of useless recipes and meal plans. I wrote this book to teach you how to make the best food choices and to teach you how to formulate your own nutritional plan.

NO ONE FOLLOWS A DIET PLAN!!! I have written thousands of nutritional plans for people over the years and no one actually follows them for more than a week. When I prescribe nutrition plans they are only samples of how to formulate a daily intake of food. I prescribe the correct food combinations and provide a variety of nutrient-dense foods to allow for different tastes. We all have to eat on a daily basis and I provide the methods to teach you how to eat according to the natural laws of human physiology. In order to be successful in changing the way you look and feel YOU MUST TAKE INVENTORY OF YOUR OWN SELF. The only one that has control of what goes into your body is YOU! I have given you my guidelines on how to eat, when to eat, and what types of food to eat. It is up to you to make the right choice.

### Eating Out

No matter where you go to eat, it is up to you to make the right decision about the best choice of food to consume. You can go anywhere and still eat within the rules of proper nutrition. First, look on the menu for the best source of protein. Next look for the best complex, water soluble vegetable. Avoid starches and ask for double vegetables if that option is available. The fat is usually in the protein source because they go hand in hand. Order a salad with salad dressing on the side. Avoid eating the bread that is usually served before your eat. Eating the bread will increase your appetite so that you will order more food. Also, too many carbohydrates will alert the sugar radar. Don't order alcoholic beverages or soda with your meal. A glass of water with lemon in it is sufficient. Avoid dessert! If you absolutely have to eat dessert, have only one to two bites. This amount is just enough to satisfy your sweet tooth.

### Eating When Coming Home From A Long, Stressful Day at the Office

Often we succumb to overeating during periods of stress. I call this *stress eating*. Stress eating is when a person is strung out from working all day and probably didn't eat much during the day. When they get home it becomes a feeding frenzy. The need for sugar is intense and the person usually scavenges through the cupboards to consume as many carbohydrates as they can find. It is very easy to consume large amounts of simple carbohydrates in a short amount of time. Having a lot of processed foods in the cupboards (cookies, pastries, candy, ice cream, chips) is dangerous for someone who is not disciplined with healthy eating or with controlling their emotions. Binge eating produces ill effects, such as: increased fat storage, poor digestion, increased production of cortisol, and negatively affects hunger hormones.

My suggestion for controlling the need to indulge in stress eating is to drink a glass of water as soon as you enter the kitchen. This will temporarily stop the sugar craving and allow time for you to prepare a protein meal. Eating sugar when you are craving sugar is counterproductive. Eating protein instead will keep your blood sugar in balance and allow you to de-stress your system without having to over-consume high glycemic foods.

## The Struggle From Within: Emotional Eating

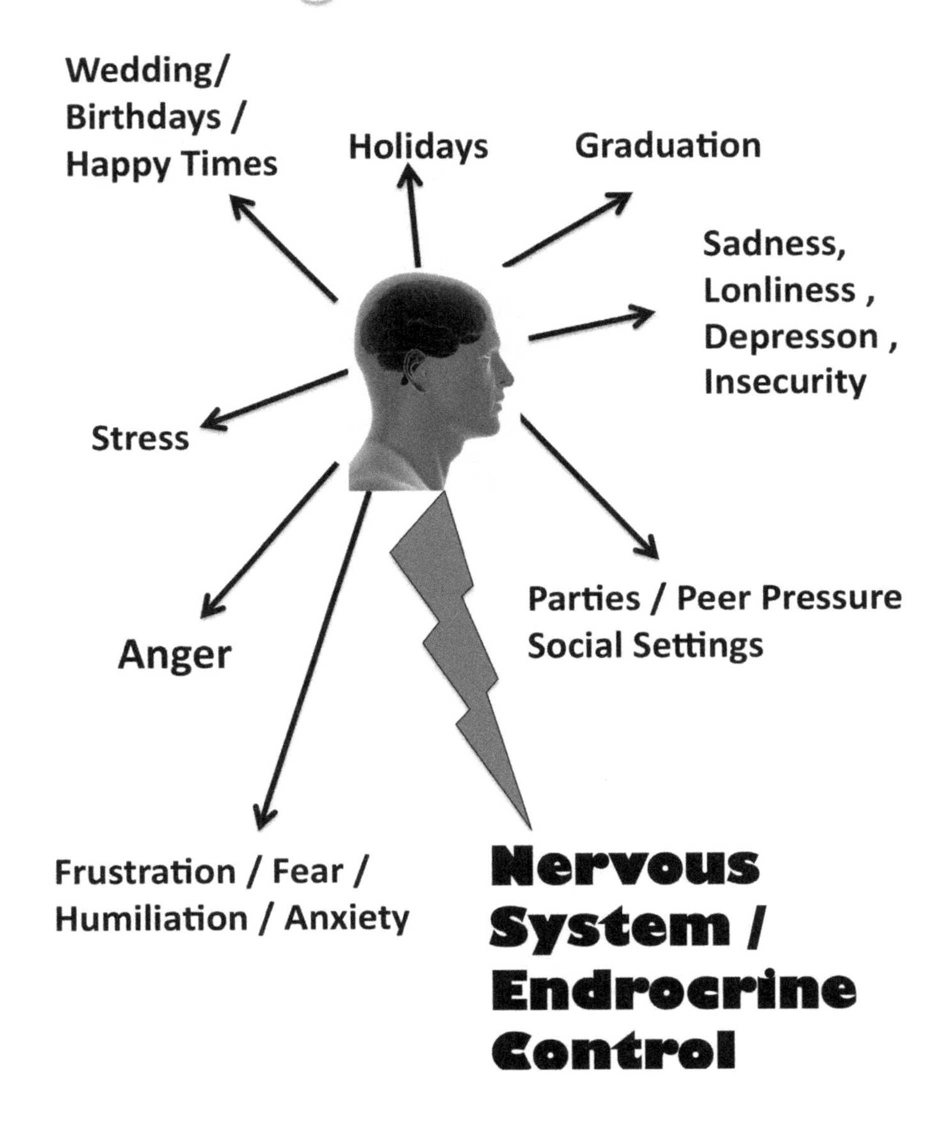


*Three of the greatest moments of my life were the birth of my two sons and daughter. Being there to see them enter into this world for the first time was splendor in the highest degree. Words cannot explain the emotion I felt inside. It was quite spiritual. My wife was amazing through it all. She is truly the strength of the family. The pain she went through is more than I could ever imagine. She was so strong and brave through the whole experience. She is a remarkable woman. I am truly her greatest fan. I love you, Joy.*

The day we were born we became attached to sugar molecules. From the moment we are expelled from the comfort of the womb we are instinctually fixated to our mother's breast milk for nourishment. Breast milk is a glucose, fat, and protein mixture that supplies the new born all the vital nutrients it needs to continue cell division and proper growth. As soon as the glucose enters the baby's mouth it stimulates the brain. The nervous system develops a link between emotion and glucose right from the start.

When the infant comes out of its mother it is terrified. This traumatic experience causes the heart rate to increase and the nervous system to react, which causes the baby to cry. The crying helps clear the lungs of amniotic fluid and other materials, as well as notify the mother that the baby is in need of something: food. Once the newborn baby attaches itself on the nipple of the mother the stress subsides. Heart rate regulates and breathing patterns stabilize. The brain makes the connection with food and emotion, this pattern is instinctual in nature. Without an intense desire to eat, infants wouldn't survive, thus civilizations wouldn't survive. Our creator knew what would be powerful enough to keep human survival going for thousands and thousands of years and that is *glucose*.

For the next few months, the only concern for the baby is physiological gratification. Sleeping, eating and eliminating seem to be the cycle of a typical day in the life of a baby. When the baby cries it receives breast milk or formula. Within seconds the crying ceases and the baby is calm. This pattern of discomfort and comfort is the cornerstone of our existence. When we are in pain we want immediate relief. Once the pain is relieved we feel better.

When the baby turns one year old it is marked by a grand celebration. Family members and friends gather to rejoice in the first year of the child's life. Food and gifts are brought and given to the baby. Everything about the birthday is happy and fun. Cake and ice cream becomes the staple of the party. Though the baby hasn't yet developed the cognitive intellect to know what is going on, it does develop a subliminal decoding of signals connected with the happy feelings associated with a party. This information is then stored in the long term memory banks of the brain for later use.

As children grow up, they begin to associate good behavior and achievements with rewards. A celebration or joyous occasion always has positive rewards attached to it.

Here are some American rituals that are celebrated with sweets, alcohol and junk food.

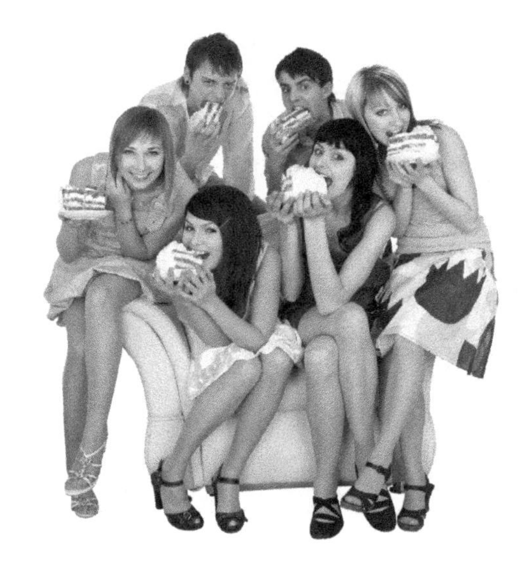

- Birthdays
- Holidays
- Good grades on a report card
- Sweet sixteen parties
- High school/college graduations
- Weddings
- 21st birthday
- A new job
- A raise or a promotion
- Coffee hour after church
- Valentines Day

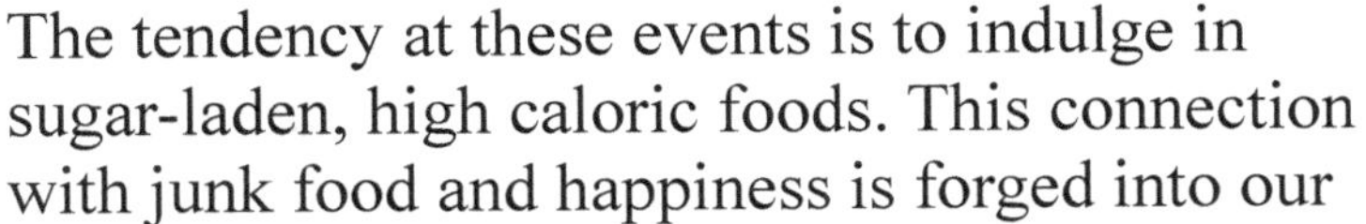

The tendency at these events is to indulge in sugar-laden, high caloric foods. This connection with junk food and happiness is forged into our subconscious throughout our lifetime. As Americans, we accept this and continue to follow the pattern from generation to generation. Celebrations are joyous occasions. However, when an individual goes through a difficult time, the need for stimulation increases. If the individual is sad, depressed, anxious, or angry brain glucose level runs low. The brain then needs more glucose and therefore recalls foods that contain simple sugars. Foods that have been consumed during celebrations tend to be recalled the fastest. This is because we have associated happiness with eating junk food. The subconscious mind remembers this, creating a tendency towards junk food in order to mimic feelings we get from being at a celebration.

When we think of a happy memory, our brain cells actually turn on the way they did during the past event, releasing the same hormonal sequence. Blood pressure changes and the heart rate slows down causing us to feel calm and content. The brain will recall these happy times when an individual becomes depressed, fearful, anxious, bored, or lonely.

When we are alone and feeling depressed or anxious the brain calls up happy memories, creating an intense desire to eat sugar. Once the sugar enters the mouth and hits the receptors in the front of the tongue the brain sets off the same neuronal pattern associated with the memory. Within minutes the fear, anxiety and depression are temporarily resolved, only to return again once the false serotonin boost ends. Our brain utilizes past memories and feelings to get what it craves--*sugar.*

When there is conflict or a threat to our survival we become angry, sad, anxious, excited, scared, and/or frustrated. Our homeostatic processes shift into a sympathetic response. To resolve the conflict the sympathetic nervous system response must be reduced. Eating food helps to resolve conflict. This pattern gets ingrained into our psyche as we live on Earth. The more we are stressed, the more we crave sugar. This pattern is why obesity is so rampant in America. Many Americans are under a tremendous amount of stress (financially, emotionally, physically) and become emotional eaters and drinkers.

Not all emotional eating is due to fear, anxiety, or depression. It can also be associated with feelings of nostalgia. Whenever I smell coffee brewing, I am instantly transported back to my grandmother's house and the many happy memories I had there. Coffee is the trigger to that memory. I don't drink coffee, but I like the smell of it. We have many triggers like this that are set up by smells and tastes. Some people like the comfort that smells and tastes of food bring to them. I have had people tell me that they don't really want to eat the donuts but the taste makes them feel like a kid again. I thought that this was very interesting. This connection is very powerful and hard to break from. I certainly can't blame a person for wanting to embrace those nostalgic feelings.

There is a powerful connection between emotions and food and for this reason people cannot be on a "diet." A diet is a way of controlling the food a person eats. Most of the time there are not enough comfort foods on a diet to satisfy the emotional state of the person. When a person's emotional state is challenged the cravings begin to increase. The crisis causes the subconscious coding to force the neurons to fire off memories and feelings attached to sugar to calm the brain. The need to feed the system becomes so powerful that the people break their restrictive diet to indulge in their addictions.

Comfort foods are instilled in the body from the moment of birth, making it hard to break the connection. Unless you are a very disciplined person who can break the subliminal coding sequences and never indulge in comfort foods, chances are you will have to have a certain amount of comfort foods in your nutritional plan to maintain balance. Donuts, pastries, coffee, cake, cookies, chocolate, ice cream, cereal, bread, beer, and wine are all examples of comfort foods. These foods are typically found at most parties and celebrations. They become engrained in the subconscious. When the need arises during a stressful event, the brain will recall these foods and force the body to go into a craving mode. I realize not everyone reading this book will give up certain comfort foods. If you need to indulge in comfort foods for balance then that is your choice, just be careful not to over do it.

# Daryl's Tongue Theory: Controlling Obesity

The tongue has taste buds. A taste bud is an area on the tongue, soft palate, upper esophagus, or epiglottis that produces taste. Taste buds identify certain types of foods as being bitter, sour, salty or sweet. The sides of the tongue respond to sour foods. The front of the tongue responds to salt and sugary foods. While the back of the tongue responds to bitter foods. These areas have receptors and nerves that when activated send a signal to the cerebral cortex of the brain. The brain then sends a signal to the stomach letting it know that food is coming. This sequence of events is also controlled by hormone secretions, especially hunger hormones. There is a direct correlation between human emotion and eating. Each area of the tongue sets off a different reaction in the brain. Sour and bitter foods tend to produce a negative effect, resulting in the individual eating less of those types of foods. Salty and sugary foods tend to produce a positive drug like feeling in the brain when those taste buds are stimulated. This is why people consume so many carbohydrates. The sugar taste buds are very sensitive and elicit an almost immediate neuronal charge in the brain. This feeling is addicting! When the endocrine system is turned on and hormones (serotonin, epinephrine, and norepinephrine) are released, brain neurons are stimulated causing a euphoric feeling. In this state pain is temporarily relieved. Pain is not limited to physical discomfort but is also associated with psychological imbalances (depression, anger, anxiety, distress, fear, sadness, loneliness, anguish).

The tongue is where obesity starts. The subconscious records and stores the sensations drawn by the sugar taste buds and will recall them during times of distress or emotional imbalance. As long as there is a connection between emotion and food it is hard to turn off this sequence of events. I feel that in order to reduce obesity the sugar taste buds need to be turned off. Many obese people resort to gastric bypass surgery or stomach stapling to control their weight. I don't believe that this is the solution. It all starts at the tongue. Most overeaters and junk food addicts only eat to satisfy the taste buds and nerves in the mouth and upper esophagus. They become addicted to receiving the "drug like" state from the sugar. Once the food enters into the stomach the effect is gone, so they continue to eat more sugar to keep the nerves firing and the brain stimulated. Once the effect reaches a point where they can no longer fit any more food into the stomach they stop eating. However, once the stomach empties the food, the process will start again from the need to consume more carbohydrates. It is a never-ending cycle for many obese people.

It is my belief that as long as the sugar receptors in the tongue are not activated, sugar cravings will reduce. Perhaps the solution to obesity is to find a way to dull the sugar taste buds. In doing this there would be no taste associated with the junk food and the desire to eat the food would decrease, thereby reducing over- consuming of junk food.

Eating foods that are low on the glycemic index activate the other areas of the tongue other than the sugar taste buds. These are the best foods to consume because they help control appetite and sugar metabolism.

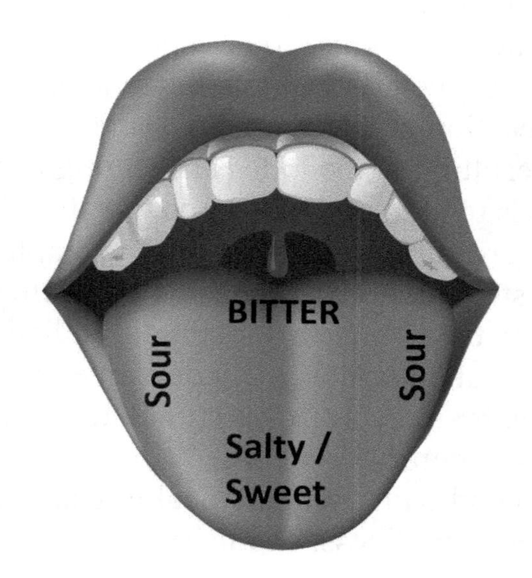

# Stress and Nutrition

We all have to deal with stress in our life. There is no getting around it. How we handle stress is the important factor for determining how our body reacts. There are two types of stress: *eustress* and *distress.*

**Eustress** is desirable stress. Exercising, laughing, sexual intercourse, amusement park rides, and playing sports are all examples of eustress. These events produce a sympathetic (fight or flight) reaction in the body. There is a change in blood pressure, sugar metabolism, oxygen uptake, and hormone secretions. Eustress actually promotes a boost in the good hormones of the body, which helps enhance the immune system. Eustress is good stress. Engaging in eustress can promote greater health. It enhances the immune system because of the release of endorphins and enkephalins in the bloodstream. These are opiate, like chemicals that help reduce pain in the body and boost immunity.

**Distress** is the undesirable stress. Sleep deprivation, worrying, anxiety, fear, hate, anger, relationship problems, physical and emotional abuse are examples of distress. When the body is in a distressed state the body systems are alerted. The sympathetic system turns on just like it does in an eustress state; however, it doesn't turn off. Eustress usually activates the sympathetic nervous system in short durations. However, when the stress lasts longer than 20-30 minutes, the body goes into distress. The more chronic the distress becomes the more the immune system is compromised. During chronic distress the body releases stress hormones to try to turn off the reaction. If the distress is not resolved, stress chemicals increase in the blood. When stress hormones epinephrine and norepinephrine are released in the blood, sugar cravings increase. This is why so many folks eat carbohydrates when they are distressed. Stress hormones trigger the release of glucose from energy stores and increases blood flow to skeletal muscle tissue. This inadvertently will increase the production of internal cholesterol levels. Once the sugar is depleted from the liver and muscle tissue, cortisol is released to help inhibit cellular permeability. When cortisol levels increase free radical production also increases. Free radicals are invaders that weaken the immune system. Vitamin and mineral concentrations also deplete during times of distress. Chronic distress will eventually decrease the immune system to the point where illness and disease can develop.

To avoid the results of distress, it is important to "de-stress" your life. Spend more time engaging in eustress and less time in distress.

Here are some ways to de-stress your life:

- **Exercise**
    - 15-45 minutes in duration
    - 3-5 times per week
    - 60-85% intensity. 85-100% if an advanced fitness participant
    - Perform both weight training and cardiovascular exercises

- **Sleep**
    - 6-8 hours is optimal

- **Power Naps**
    - Take a 5-15 minute nap during the day to re-energize.

- **Deep Breathing Techniques**
    - Meditation
    - Yoga or similar type of exercise
    - Diaphragmatic Breathing. Deep breathing focusing on getting all the air out of the diaphragm

- **Develop a Hobby**
    - Learn a new skill
    - Take up painting
    - Gardening

- **Walk a Dog**
- **Go on a Vacation**
- **Go Hiking**
- **Play Golf**
- **Learn How To Play Tennis**
- **Swim**
- **Take Walk Around The Neighborhood**

# Designing Your Daily Food Intake

The key to eating healthy, is to choose the best sources of nutrients you can find anywhere you go. If the only place I could eat was McDonalds, then I would try to find the best nutrients they had, even while realizing that there wouldn't be many. But if my life depended on it I would make the best out of it. When I go to a restaurant, the first thing I look for on the menu is the best source of protein,which is usually filet mignon. Then I will search for the best water soluble vegetable to accompanying the beef, which is most of the time broccoli or spinach. I will also have a salad with dressing on the side. I take a couple digestive enzymes and supplements (amino acids, multivitamins, etc.) before I eat and that is it. No matter where I go, I will try to make the best food choice. If you think of protein first, fat second, and carbohydrates last you will be better off. I want you to count protein grams rather than calories. The body can only digest roughly thirty grams of protein every couple of hours. The excess protein above thirty grams will most likely be converted to sugar or eliminated out of the body, never to be utilized. The formula I have developed is simple. After awhile you won't have to write anything down because you will know how to choose the right foods and the right amount each time you eat. It will become natural to you.

**Here Are My Rules For Eating (Recap)**

- Eat 5-6 small meals a day
- Eat every 2-3 hours (grazing)
- Count protein grams per meal
- Count sugar grams, keeping intake low. Try to eat low glycemic carbs.
- Follow the food combining rules
- Take digestive enzymes
- Take supplements
- Consume good fats (flaxseed, salmon oil)
- Don't drink lots of liquid with food
- Eat a protein as the last meal of the day
- Limit comfort foods to as minimal as possible
- Don't drink alcohol
- Don't smoke cigarettes
- Put feet up after eating
- Chew food completely
- Don't engulf food
- Never add salt to food

- Pay attention to how you react from food. Increased pulse, increased blood pressure, sneezing, headache, indigestion, gas, diarrhea and/or after eating could indicate that you have allergies
- Avoid emotional eating.

Applying these simple rules will make designing your meal plan easy and effortless. The following chart is a simple way of tracking the food you eat. Once you know the amount of nutrients you are taking in per meal, over time, you won't have to write down anything because it will come to you automatically. The goal is to make this process as simple as possible. The easier it is, the more successful you will become.

**The following meal plans and supplement schedules are examples only, though these plans are accurate and safe, I recommend that you consult a professional who is educated in natural nutrition. Email me if you cannot find someone in your surrounding area. Dconant2004@yahoo.com**

**A Simple Charting of Nutrients**

It is important to write out your daily food intake to keep track of the amount of vital nutrients you are consuming. Here is a simple way to record your food intake.

**Meal 1:** **Protein**______________________________

**Fat**______________________________

**Low Glycemic Complex Carbs**______________

**Meal 2:** **Protein**______________________________

**Fat**______________________________

**Low Glycemic Complex Carbs**______________

**Meal 3:** **Protein**______________________________

**Fat**______________________________

**Low Glycemic Complex Carbs**______________

**Meal 4:** **Protein**______________________________

**Fat**______________________________

**Low Glycemic Complex Carbs**______________

**Meal 5:** **Protein**______________________________

**Fat**______________________________

**Low Glycemic Complex Carbs**______________

**Meal 6:** **Protein**______________________________

**Fat**______________________________

**Low Glycemic Complex Carbs**______________

Here is what a sample plan looks like. **SAMPLE MAINTENANCE PLAN**

**Meal 1:** **Protein** 4 Eggs Lightly Scrambled

**Fat** 1 tsp Unsalted Natural Butter / and Yolks from Eggs

**Complex Carbs** 2 oz. Raw Natural Organic Spinach

**Meal 2:** **Protein** 1 Cup Cottage Cheese

**Fat** Cottage Cheese and 1 Flax Seed Tablet

**Complex Carbs** Lactose in Cottage Cheese

**Meal 3:** **Protein** 6 oz. Flank Steak

**Fat** Saturated Fat From Steak/ 1 Fish Oil Tablet/ 1 tsp. Olive oil

**Complex Carbs** 4 oz. Green Leafy Vegetables / Olive Oil Vinegar Dressing

**Meal 4:** **Protein** 2 oz. Raw Cheddar Cheese

**Fat** Saturated Fat

**Complex Carbs** Lactose in Cheese

**Meal 5:** **Protein** 6 oz. Salmon

**Fat** Omega-3 from Salmon

**Complex Carbs** 1 cup Steamed Broccoli

**Meal 6:** **Protein** 20 Non-Salted Almonds

**Fat** Alpha Lineoliec Acid in Almonds

**Complex Carbs** Fiber in Almonds

** Supplements to be taken with maintenance plan:

*Continued*

Digestive Enzymes
Free Form Amino Acids
Dessicated Liver Tablets
Branched Chain Amino Acids
Fish Oil
Flax Seed Oil
Essential Minerals
Time Released Multi-Vitamin Pack
Glandulars
Vitamin C
Zinc

**Supplement schedule for the day**

**Upon waking on empty stomach**
6 Free Form Amino Acid Tablets

**Before breakfast**
Time Released Multi-vitamin Pack
2-4 Digestive Enzymes
1 Fish Oil

**Immediately following breakfast**
6-10 Dessicated Liver Tablets
2-6 Glandulars

**In between breakfast and lunch**
4-6 Free Form Amino Acids
2-6 Dessicated Liver Tablets

**Before lunch**
2-4 Digestive enzymes
1 Flax Seed Tablet

**Immediately following lunch**
6-10 Dessicated Liver Tablets
2-6 Glandulars

*Continued*

**In between lunch and dinner**

4-6 Free Form Amino Acids
2-6 Dessicated Liver Tablets

**Before Dinner**

2-4 Digestive Enzymes
1 Fish oil
2 Essential Minerals
1 Vitamin C
1 Zinc

**Immediately following dinner**

6-10 Dessicated Liver Tablets
4-6 Free Form Amino Acids

Please note: This meal plan sample is not to be followed verbatim. The intake of protein, fats, and carbohydrates vary from person to person. You have to figure your own intake requirement. Refer back to page 82 for the formula of figuring out your protein intake.

Here is what a sample plan looks like. **SAMPLE MUSCLE BUILDING PLAN**

**Meal 1:** **Protein** 4 Eggs Lightly Scrambled Mixed in 1 tbsp. Sour Cream

**Fat** 1 tbsp Unsalted Natural Butter / and Yolks from Eggs/ Sour cream

**Complex Carbs** 2 oz. Raw Natural Organic Spinach

**Meal 2:** **Protein** Protein Drink Powder,1/2 and 1/2 Cream

**Fat** Cream/ Egg Yolks

**Complex Carbs** None

**Meal 3:** **Protein** 30 Grams of. Flank Steak/ Filet Mignon

**Fat** Saturated Fat from Steak

**Complex Carbs** 4 oz. Green Leafy Vegetables / Olive Oil Vinegar Dressing

**Meal 4:** **Protein** Protein Drink Same as Meal 2

**Fat** Same

**Complex Carbs** Same

**Meal 5:** **Protein** 30 Grams of Meat

**Fat** From Meat

**Complex Carbs** 1 Cup Steamed Broccoli

**Meal 6:** **Protein** Protein Drink Same as Meal 2 and 4

**Fat** Same

**Complex Carbs** Trace Amount in Protein Powder

Eat every 72 hours a complex carbohydrate meal to fill glycogen stores.

Suggestions:

You can choose one of the following for your carbohydrate meal. Eat no protein with this meal.

- Whole wheat pasta
- A baked potato with sour cream
- A big salad with many vegetables
- Bowl of oatmeal
- Yam
- Fruit

**Supplements schedule for the day:**

**Upon waking on empty stomach**

6 Free Form Amino Acid Tablets

**Before breakfast**

Time Released Multi-vitamin Pack
2-4 Digestive Enzymes
1 Fish Oil
4 Free Form Amino Acid Tablets
2-6 Dessicated Liver Tablets

**Immediately following breakfast**

6-10 Dessicated Liver Tablets
2-6 Glandulars

**In between breakfast and lunch**

4-6 Free Form Amino Acids
2-6 Dessicated Liver Tablets

**Before Lunch**

2-4 Digestive enzymes
1 Flax Seed Tablet
4 Free Form Amino Acid Tablets
2-6 Dessicated Liver Tablets

*continued*

**Immediately following lunch**

6-10 Dessicated Liver Tablets
2-6 Glandulars

**In between lunch and dinner**

4-6 Free Form Amino Acids
2-6 Dessicated Liver Tablets

**Before dinner**

2-4 Digestive Enzymes
1 Fish oil
2 Essential Minerals
1 Vitamin C
1 Zinc
4 Free Form Amino Acids

**Immediately following dinner**

6-10 Dessicated Liver Tablets
4-6 Free Form Amino Acids

**An hour before working out**

2-4 Orchic Tablets
6-10 Dessicated Liver Tablets
6-10 Branched Chain Aminos

**30 Minutes after Post Workout Protein Shake**

6-10 Branched Chain Aminos

**Before retiring:** 30 minutes before sleep

2 L-Glycine Tablets

**Please note: This meal plan sample is not to be followed verbatim. The intake of protein, fats, and carbohydrates vary from person to person. You have to figure your own intake requirement.**

Here is what a sample plan looks like. SAMPLE **THE LAZY BASTARD**

I realize that not everyone is going to follow the maintenance or muscle building plans that I have outlined previously. Here is a plan for even the most non-disciplined person in the world-- "The Lazy Bastard."

The same rules apply as with the other meal plans except there are no supplements. I do not even put in the digestive enzymes because the Lazy Bastard does not have the patience or discipline to take them on a daily basis.

Here is what a sample plan looks like. **The LAZY BASTARD PLAN**

**Meal 1:** **Protein** 2 or 4 Eggs Scrambled

**Fat** 1 tbsp. Butter for Cooking, 1 tbsp Butter for Toast

**Low Glycemic Complex Carbs** 1-2 Pieces Whole Wheat Toast

**Meal 2:** **Protein** Natural Yogurt

**Fat** Saturated Fat In Yogurt

**Low Glycemic Complex Carbs** Lactose in Yogurt

**Meal 3:** **Protein** 6-8 ounces of Chicken

**Fat** Olive Oil Dressing

**Low Glycemic Complex Carbs** Salad with Vegetables

**Meal 4:** **Protein** Almond Butter

**Fat** Alpha Lineoliec Acid in Almonds

**Moderate Glycemic Complex Carbs** Apple

**Meal 5:** **Protein** 10 ounce Steak

**Fat** Saturated fat from steak

**Low Glycemic Complex Carbs** Salad with Vegetables

**Meal 6**: **Protein** 2 Cups of Milk

**Fat** Saturated Fat in Milk

**Low Glycemic Complex Carbs** Lactose in milk

Here is what a sample plan looks like. **SAMPLE FAT LOSS PLAN**

**Meal 1:** **Protein** 2-4 Eggs Lightly Scrambled

**Fat** 1 tbsp Unsalted Natural Butter / and Yolks from Eggs

**Complex Carbs** 2 oz. Raw Natural Organic Spinach

**Meal 2:** **Protein** 1 Cup Cottage Cheese

**Fat** Cottage Cheese and 1 Flax Seed Tablet

**Complex Carbs** Lactose in Cottage Cheese

**Meal 3:** **Protein** NONE

**Fat** 2 tbsp. Olive oil / Vinegar Dressing

**Complex Carbs** Super Salad: A Variety of Raw Vegetables, Spinach, Green Leafy Vegetables, Broccoli

**Meal 4:** **Protein** 2 oz. Raw Cheddar Cheese

**Fat** Saturated Fat in Cheddar Cheese

**Complex Carbs** Lactose in Cheese

**Meal 5:** **Protein** 6 oz. Organic Chicken Baked

**Fat** Chicken Fat

**Complex Carbs** 1 cup Steamed Broccoli

**Meal 6:** **Protein** 20 Non-Salted Almonds

**Fat** Alpha Lineoliec Acid in Almonds

**Complex Carbs** Fiber in Almonds

**Supplement schedule for the day**
Upon waking on empty stomach.
- 6 Free Form Amino Acid Tablets

**Before breakfast**
- Time Released Multi-vitamin Pack
- 2-3 Fat Burners
- 2-4 Digestive Enzymes
- 1 Fish Oil

**Immediately following breakfast**
- 6-10 Dessicated Liver Tablets
- 2-6 Glandulars

**In between breakfast and lunch**
- 4-6 Free Form Amino Acids
- 2-6 Dessicated Liver Tablets

**Before lunch**
- 2-3 Fat Burners
- 4 Branched Chain Amino Acids
- 2-4 Digestive enzymes
- 1 Flax Seed Tablet

**Immediately following Lunch**
- 6-10 Dessicated Liver Tablets
- 2-6 Glandulars

**In between lunch and dinner**
- 4-6 Free Form Amino Acids
- 2-6 Dessicated Liver Tablets

**Before dinner**
- 2-3 Fat Burners
- 2-4 Digestive Enzymes
- 1 Fish oil
- 2 Essential Minerals
- 1 Vitamin C
- 1 Zinc

**Immediately following dinner**
6-10 Dessicated Liver Tablets
4-6 Free Form Amino Acids

**During Workout**
1 Tbsp. Liquid L-Carnitine In 8 oz. Of Water. Sip throughout the workout.

**NOTE:**
**The previous meal <u>templates are only samples</u> to show how a meal plan looks like. Now I would like to explain how to design a sensible plan for your self.**

Using the nutrient chart, simply plug in your food choices.

1. Figure out your daily protein requirement.
The appropriate amount of dietary protein is as follows;
sedentary adult .8 x BW(body weight) = Daily Required Intake (DRI), active adult 1 x BW = DRI, Athlete 1.2 x BW= DRI.

2. Always write down the essential fat grams.

3. Write down the low glycemic low carbohydrate food. The amount to take in depends on the sugar content. You can eat more of the low glycemic foods because the sugar radar won't be activated.

4. Make sure that the combinations of food fall into the correct criteria of food combining.

5. Take the appropriate supplements.

**It is very easy once you begin to identify to the foods you eat. This process should not be labor intensive.**

The supplements listed are the ones that I use and recommend. I have provided a complete list of many commonly used supplements in Appendix II. You can decide which ones are best for you. Everyone's needs are different.

# How Much Should You Eat Per Feeding?

One of the greatest pitfalls with eating is consuming too much food per feeding. Over-consuming food puts too much stress on the digestive system. As discussed earlier, when the digestive system is compromised, nutrient exchange is poor. In order to optimize nutrient uptake eating smaller amounts of food is the key.

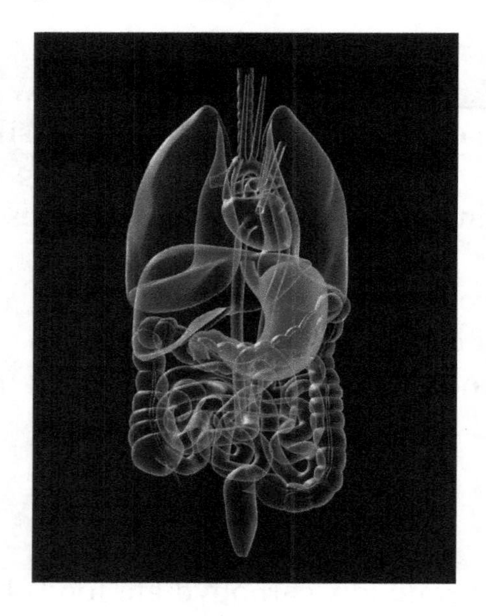

Rather than getting too bogged down with measuring everything you eat with a scale, I recommend using your hand as a guide. Your stomach is about as big as your hand. To keep the stomach its regular size it is important not to overeat. The stomach can handle excess consumption every now and again. However, if over consumption is chronic, then the stomach will eventually stretch to accommodate for the amount of food that has entered.

The stomach has nerves attached to its lining. When the stomach is empty the afferent nerves send a signal to the brain. The brain then activates hunger hormones to stimulate appetite. The person then eats. When the stomach is full, the lining becomes taut. This tautness stimulates the afferent nerves to send another signal to the brain to release hormones to stop the feeding cycle. If the stomach is not filled enough to cause a tautness of the lining, the neural signal is inhibited. Therefore, the feeding sequence continues.

When the stomach is constantly being forced to take in more food than it can handle, it will stretch to accommodate for the excess food. Now, every time food is delivered to the stomach it must be in the same amount as before in order to make the stomach taut. Otherwise the brain will not turn off the eating cycle. Chronic overeating will cause a distended stomach and stretched intestines.

Reducing the size of the stomach and intestines starts with eating small meals about the size of your hand. This is all the food the body needs to sustain the VNES every couple of hours. By keeping the amount of food small, the stomach will become taut with less food, which will allow the afferent nerves to signal the brain to stop eating. The stomach learns to adapt to the amount of food that is being delivered. If you have an enlarged stomach due to overeating, the stomach can shrink to a smaller size over a period of time if you stick to eating small meals.

**The Omentum**

The *omentum* is a large fold of tissue that hangs down from the stomach. It is a storage sack of fat. There are two sections of the omentum, the greater and the lesser. The greater sits in front of the stomach, and the lesser sits in front of the liver. The purpose of the omentum is to store excess fat that the stomach and intestines have not yet digested. It is a temporary holding depot. The size of the omentum can get very large from chronic overeating. The omentum not only stores excess fat but also stores the stress hormone cortisol. Cortisol is released when the body is under stress. The more stress a person is under the larger the omentum becomes. A large distended omentum puts the heart and arteries at risk for developing disease. Eating small, nutrient-dense meals, reducing stress and exercising on a regular basis will help shrink an over-enlarged omentum.

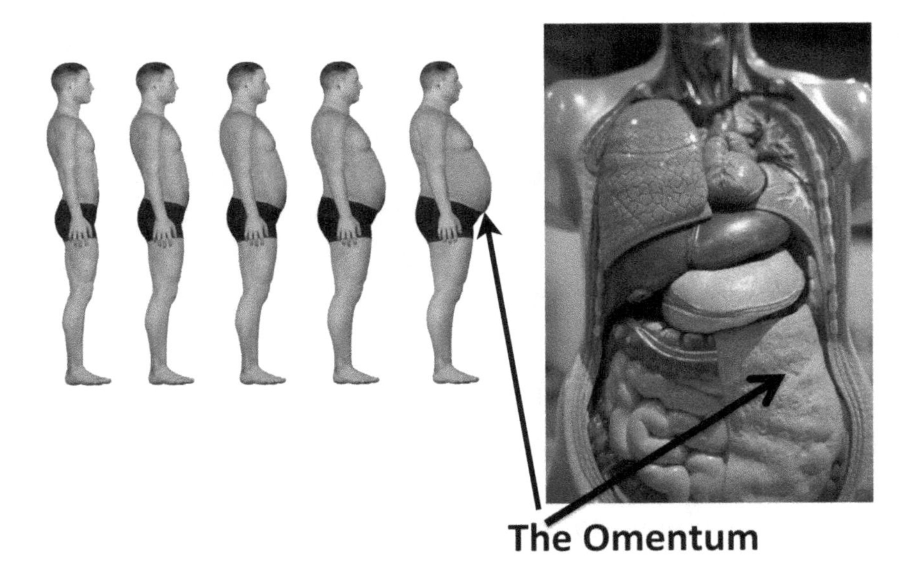

The Omentum

## Discipline

The number one reason why a person fails to achieve the body that they desire is lack of discipline. Many people eat terribly and then exercise to make up for their nutritional sins. This never works! Proper nutrition is not a temporary fix, it is a lifestyle commitment. I have little tolerance for people who complain about eating vegetables or protein. Those that really want to see a change will do whatever it takes to do so. When I was in my teens I was told to eat broccoli because it was a great food with lots of nutrients. I didn't like it for many years, but I ate it because I knew of the benefits. I became very disciplined at an early age and it has paid off. Discipline is something you can not teach. You either have it or you don't. People who are constantly fluctuating in weight are incapable of staying disciplined. I do not eat food for comfort or for taste. I eat food solely for the purpose of supplying my body with the nutrients required for building and repairing cells. I realize not everyone is like this. I don't expect people to eat like I do, or to follow everything I say. I like the benefits I get from eating healthy. It is up to you to discover what works best. I have presented methods on how to eat and how to develop your own meal plans. It is up to you to take what you have learned and better yourself through healthy eating.

### Geographical Eating

When people go to Florida in the winter they often times come back to New England and catch a cold. They also bring back with them fresh oranges and grape fruits. I began to analyze why people get sick when coming home from warmer climates during the winter months. Going on a vacation would seem to be a relaxing event. Most people go on vacation to rid the stress in their life and to take a break from the grind. Yet, many people who go to a warm environment during the winter months end up catching a cold when they come home. After analyzing this phenomenon I have come up with my own theory as to why these people get sick.

I have lived in New England the majority of my life. During the year, New Englanders experience a change in seasons. Spring, Summer, Fall, and Winter are four distinct seasons in New England. There is a distinct change in climate during the four seasons. During Fall the trees begin to lose their leaves and the sun begins to get further away, reducing the amount of sunlight. This reduction in sunlight begins to decrease serotonin levels in the human body. The blood begins to change into a more viscous substance to prepare the body for the "hibernation" phase. The hibernation phase occur during the winter months. Animals in cold climates tend to sleep more and crave storing fuel for the long months ahead. Though we don't sleep for months like our ancestors did or like bears do, humans today still gravitate toward storing fuel and sleeping for longer than normal periods during the winter months. There is also a direct connection with psychological well being during the hibernation months. Many people are affected by lack of sunlight. They might become Vitamin D deficient and develop deep depression. The depression is related to low levels of serotonin. During the winter months the brain releases less serotonin, making the central nervous system depressed. Hormone production is altered and sugar metabolism increases. Folks who suffer from prolonged depression during the cold months are thought to have SAD (seasonal affective disorder). There is a direct correlation to lack of sunlight and a person's mood.

The blood systems of animals adapts to the changes in climate. In cold weather, the blood becomes more viscous to conserve nutrients and body heat. During winter, animals, tend to hibernate. The hibernation phase is innate in all cold weather mammals. When Spring returns, the body slowly comes out of the hibernative state and starts to increase hormone production. This is why so many animals mate during the spring months as there is a surge in reproductive hormones. Serotonin levels increase and the sunlight becomes stronger and lasts longer during the day. The sun provides Vitamin D and this helps nourish and energizes the body. During the summer months, the blood becomes less viscous to help cool the body and to help move nutrients through the body faster. Also, less sleep is needed during the summer. The body is directly affected by the changing seasons. There is a distinct change in hormone levels, blood pressure, and the circulatory system, during the different seasons.

Before the advances of transportation, humans were subjected to staying in their geographical regions throughout the seasons. Now we have airplanes, trains, and cars that can transport us from a cold to warm climate within a couple of hours or days. Here is my theory on why people may become sick during the winter months while visiting the warmer climates.

As I discussed, the blood system acclimates to varying weather changes. Now when a person in the northern part of the country goes away on a vacation, they usually pick the darkest, coldest time of year -- January or February. This means that they have been acclimated to a cold environment for a couple of months already. Their blood system has become more viscous. Now they get on a plane and are in a tropical climate within 2-6 hours. Their body is not ready for such a drastic change in climate and this forces the immune system to become compromised. Eventually the blood system will adapt to the new climate change. Usually by the end of the week the hormone levels begin to increase like they would in the spring and summer months. However, this is only a temporary hormone boost. The person now has to travel back home to the cold weather climate. Their blood has become thinner and now they don't have the protection against the cold as they did when they acclimated to the climate change. The immune system defense is compromised, which may lead to catching a cold.

How does this relate to nutrition? I believe that we should only eat foods within a particular geographical region. If people from the north were supposed to eat citrus fruits during the winter, then I believe that orange groves would be grown in the northern states. However, you will never see oranges growing from trees in Maine during the winter months. Citrus fruits help contribute to thinning the blood in hot climates. This could explain why we catch a cold in the winter months. We are taught that drinking orange juice is a great source of Vitamin C. Oranges are a natural blood thinner and they grow in warm climates. Drinking orange juice in colder climates can cause the blood to become thinner, making the body more susceptible to illness.

Technology has allowed us to obtain foods from all over the world in only a couple of days. However, foods that are not available in the geographical location that we live in may not be the best for us. For example pure soy protein comes from China and is their main food source. Soy protein is easy to harvest in China making it a great means of feeding the masses. The Chinese people seldom develop any side effects from eating soy protein. This is because for centuries and centuries they have developed the enzymes to digest the bean product without any adverse effects. Americans adopted soy protein as a replacement to eating animal protein. However, Americans who eat large quantities of soy protein can develop too much estrogen in the body, which can cause illness and possibly cancer.

Eating foods that we can only get in our geographical surroundings might be the best choice for maintaining a balance between nature and our health. If a food cannot be grown during a particular season, then the body does not need it. There is a reason why we don't see tropical fruit tree growing in Maine during the winter months. I feel that we should only eat the foods that are grown in our natural geographical surroundings with the exception of meats and vegetables. Meats and vegetables can be frozen and stored for months. Fruits cannot be frozen and still hold their nutritional value.

# Hormones and Aging

## Aging: Catabolic Degeneration

Aging is a natural human process. From the moment of conception the cells of the body begin to age. While in the womb the cells of the embryo replicate, split, and divide to form into a baby nine months later. The development of the embryo through mitosis and meiosis (cell division) occurs at an extremely fast rate. Cell division continues throughout our entire life. The cells of the body are constantly dying and regenerating themselves. When we are young, 0-25 years of age, respectively, our body is in a high *anabolic state.* The anabolic state is when the cells of the body replicate at a fast rate. Hormones, protein, fat, sugar synthesis, flexibility, tissue repair, and cell replication are at their greatest level of production during the anabolic years.

After the age of about 25, the body begins to go into a slow and steady *catabolic state.* A catabolic state is when the cells of the body die and are not regenerated as fast or at all. The older we get the greater the catabolic effect becomes, also known as the aging process. The catabolic state of aging is inescapable. However, there are strategies that can help reduce the catabolic process, slowing it down considerably.

There are two types of aging: *time dependent age* and *acquired age.*
***Time Dependent age*** is the normal aging processes of the body dictated by genetics, DNA Coding, and hereditary factors. Time dependent aging can be slowed down by following a healthy nutrition program, exercising, and reducing stressors.

***Acquired Age*** is caused by self-inflicted desires. Smoking, alcohol abuse, refined sugars, food preservatives, white enriched flour, hydrogenated oils, fast foods, skipping meals, stressful living, drugs, and stimulants all contribute to destroying cells of the body at a faster-than-normal rate. Acquired age is an accelerated aging effect that is brought about by an individual's habits and lifestyle. When the cells die at a faster rate than expected, the immune system is compromised and the tissues of the body begin to die faster. People who are constantly polluting their systems with junk food and narcotics end up prematurely killing their organs. An example of this occurs when a person over consumes sugar for years. The pancreas can no longer produce enough insulin to keep up with the amount of sugar being taken in by the body. Eventually the pancreas will burn out, and insulin will no longer be produced, giving rise to diabetes.

Diabetics are getting younger and younger by the day. Long ago diabetes was a rare disease but now it is becoming more prevalent. Over consumption of sugar is also attributed to the death of the arteries and the heart. Consuming too much sugar can accelerate the onset of plaque in the arteries, and can ultimately cause the heart to stop due to the lack of blood being pumped into the chambers from the blockage of plaque in the arteries. Sugar forms cracks in the lining of the arteries and tissues, causing the production of cholesterol and fat to accumulate and be stored in those areas.

Acquired age factors can cause early aging and the onset of disease. Reducing these factors can greatly reduce the inflammatory processes, therefore slowing down the aging process.

The natural processes of **time dependent aging** are responsible for the reduction of hormone levels as we age. Building muscle becomes harder when the catabolic shift begins to take over. Though we can continue to build muscle in the latter years of life, the gains might not be as significant as they were when we were young. This is because testosterone, insulin, and growth hormone concentrations decrease considerably. If you started weight training at an early age (teens, twenties) and have continued throughout your life, chances are you have a higher than normal level of testosterone in your body and might not see a dramatic loss in muscle tissue until much later in life.

Although we cannot stop the aging process entirely, we can reduce its onset. Genetics, good nutritional habits, supplements, good psychological well-being, and exercise (staying active) can all help slow down the process of aging.

One of the most noticeable effects of aging occurs to the skin. As we age the skin loses much of its elasticity and taughtness. Many people have plastic surgery to fight the effects of aging. What is happening is that the cells are decreasing at a faster rate. This is called *protein disintegration.* Cells continue to die without replication. Also, the size of the cells increase. This happens because when we were young, the cells were bountiful, and pressed together tightly to form a tight young body. As we age the cells disperse because of the extra room, so the cells spread out to accommodate the space. When the cells spread they do not have the same youthful matrix that tighter cells have. Weight training can help maintain the cells as we age. However, eventually we all succumb to the aging effect. The goal of exercise is to take the body to its maximum ability all the way to the end. I exercise to help keep my body healthy and strong. I realize I will probably be half the size I am now in my old age, with sagging wrinkled skin and white hair, but I will take this body to the limit all the way to my last breath. The more you use the body; the more you will get from it.

**Protein Disintegration (release of suspension)**

Protein is the most important element for human tissue growth. I believe that the body goes through stages of development that shift every ten years. If you notice human bodies as they age you will notice that the fat percentage increases and muscle volume decreases (atrophy). The reason for this is because of protein disintegration. Protein disintegration is when the suspension of protein releases and changes the matrix of the body. Body composition changes and the cells diminish. The goal is to try to keep active protein for as long as possible. Maintaining the appropriate amounts of protein intake on a daily basis throughout life will help keep active protein lasting longer, slowing down the aging effect. When the body does not take in the correct amount of protein externally and has to depend on catabolizing internal protein (muscle) to supply the body, this forces the break down matrix of growth factors and tissue, changing body composition. When muscle is catabolized internally, it can become anabolic again if the protein levels are brought back up from eating good sources of protein. This is why it is so important to maintain proper protein levels throughout life. The objective is to avoid catabolism and to keep protein active for as long as possible.

## Boosting Your Active Metabolism To Maximize Fat Burning

Here are a couple of exercise programs to boost your active metabolism.

**Perform:**
**1 Set For Beginner (Never exercised before)**
**2 Set For Moderate (Regular exerciser 2 times per week)**
**3 Set For Advanced (Have been exercising regularly 3 times per week)**

**12 Repetitions Per Set**

**Frequency:** Perform 3 times per week.
**Duration:** Complete each program within 30 minutes.
**Intensity:** Work at 85% maximum. To determine 85% lift a weight where you can only perform 6 reps. By the sixth rep you should not be able to do any more reps. This will be your maximum weight. Multiply the maximum weight number by .85 this will be the intensity to use for each exercise.

## Home Program:

**Program I:**

- Sit Squats
- Dumbell Press
- One Arm Row
- Seated Lateral Raise
- Seated Bicep Curl
- Tricep Kickback
- Frog Sit-Ups

**Program II:**

- Dumbell Lunges
- Dumbell Chest Fly
- Bentover Row
- Upright Row
- Standing Bicep Curl
- Tricep Bench Dips
- Abdominal Bicycle

## In The Gym: General Conditioning

***Machine Program***

- Leg Press
- Seated Hamstring Curl
- Chest Press
- Back Row
- Lat Pulldown
- Shoulder Press
- Cable Bicep Curl
- Tricep Pressdown
- Ab Bench

***Free Weight Program***

- Barbell Squat
- Ball Hamstring Tuck
- Dumbell Flat Bench Chest Press
- Lat Pulldown
- Bent Over Dumbell Row (Head on Bench)
- Seated Lateral Raise
- Barbell Bicep Curl
- Tricep Overhead Dumbell Extension
- Abdominal Plank

## In The Gym: Bone Building Emphasis

**Perform:**
**1 Set For Beginner (Never exercised before)**
**2 Set For Moderate (Regular exerciser 2 times per week)**
**3 Set For Advanced (Have been exercising regularly 3 times per week)**

**5-12 Repetitions Per Set**

**Frequency:** Perform 3 times per week.
**Duration:** Complete each program within 30 minutes.
**Intensity:** Work at 85%-95% maximum. To determine 85% lift a weight where you can only perform 6 reps. By the sixth rep you should not be able to do any more reps. This will be your maximum weight. Multiply the maximum weight number by .85 this will be the intensity to use for each exercise.

***Beginner***
- Barbell Squat
- Deadlift
- Flat Bench Barbell Chest Press

***Advanced***
- Barbell Squat
- Deadlift
- Flat Bench Barbell Chest Press
- Bent Over Barbell Row
- High Pulls
- Standing One Legged Bicep Curl
- Barbell Overhead Extension

## Functional Training Program

***Beginner***

- Clean and Press
- One Arm Single Leg Cable Pull
- Wood Chop
- Transverse Cable Rotation
- Walking Lunges
- Lateral Strides w/ Dumbell Press

***Advanced***

- Clean and Press
- One Arm Single Leg Cable Pull
- Wood Chop
- Transverse Cable Rotation
- Walking Lunges
- Lateral Strides w/ Dumbell Press
- Deadlift
- Medicine Ball Push Ups
- Medicine Ball Up Wood Chop

## Home Program:

# Program I:

- Sit Squats
- Dumbell Press
- One Arm Row
- Seated Lateral Raise
- Seated Bicep Curl
- Tricep Kickback
- Frog Sit-Ups

This program is designed for the home setting. All you need is a small dumbell set ranging from 5-12 pounds. When you become more advanced you may want to consider upgrading your dumbell set to 15-25 pounds.

Here are the exercises and instructions.

# Sit Squats

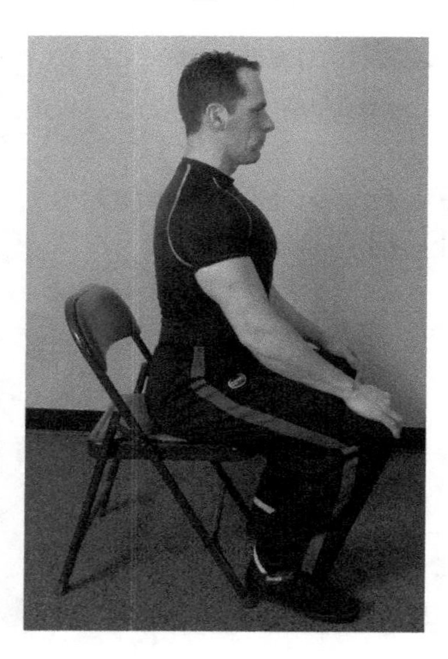

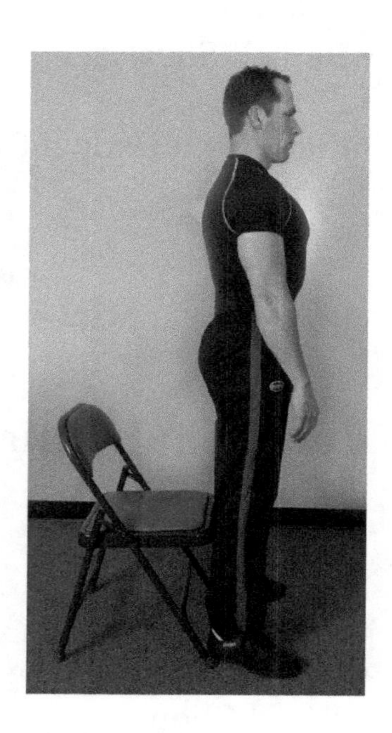

**Start** **Finish**

Sit on a chair. Keep back straight. Hands on top of legs. Feet are flat on ground shoulder width apart. Stand up hinging at the hip not the lower back. Put your weight on your legs. Tuck hips in while standing up. Repeat the sequence until all repetitions are achieved. Rest, take 6 deep breaths, then continue your next set.

# Dumbell Chest Press

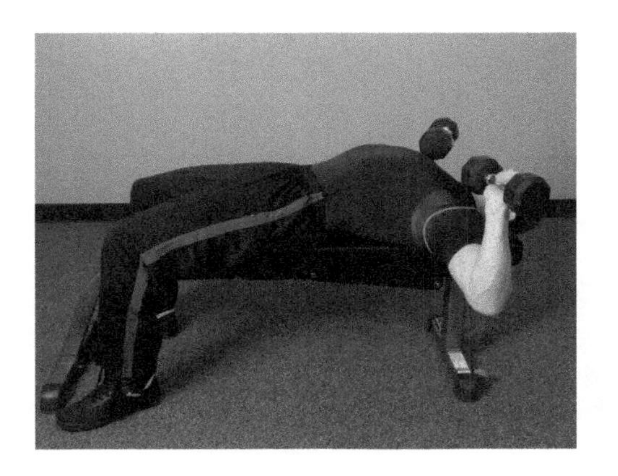

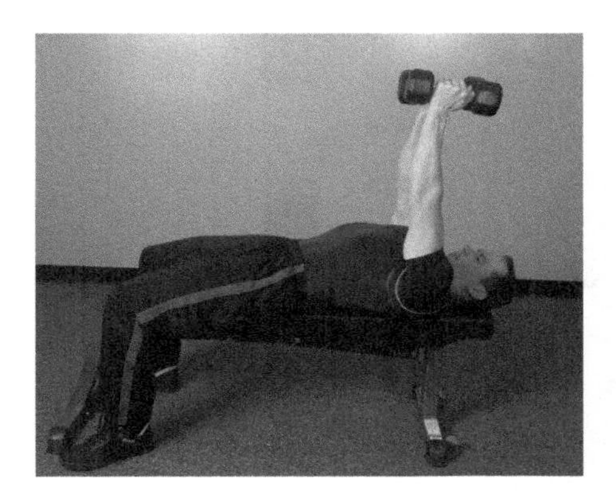

## Start

## Finish

Lying on a flat bench. If you don't have a flat bench you can lie down on the floor with bent knees and feet flat on the floor. Start with the elbows wide stretching the chest. The dumbells are aligned with the arm with palms facing feet. Exhale and push the dumbells up. Slowly turn the dumbells in on the way up, ultimately meeting at the top of the movement above the chest. Avoid extending elbows fully. A slight bend is preferable. Slowly return swinging the elbows out wide to feel the stretch in the chest. Repeat the sequence until all repetitions are achieved. Rest, take 6 deep breaths, then continue your next set.

# One Arm Dumbell Row

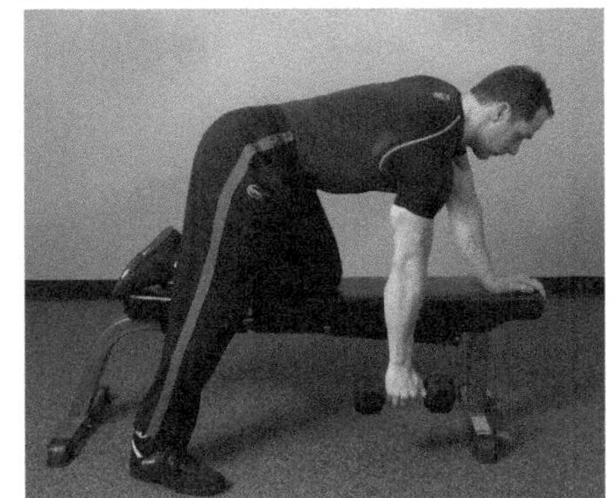

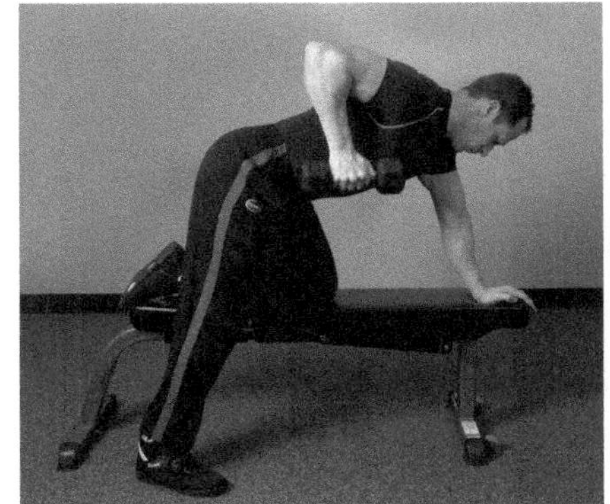

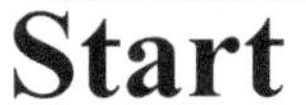

## Start

## Finish

Kneeling on a flat bench. Place one hand on the bench for support, arm extended. This helps keep the back straight. Start with a dumbell in the other hand, arm extended. Raise dumbell up toward the side of your body squeezing the back tightly into contraction. Avoid rotating the hip, keep the back still. Slowly return the weight into the starting position. Repeat the sequence until all repetitions are achieved. Rest, take 6 deep breaths, then continue your next set.

# Seated Dumbell Lateral Raise

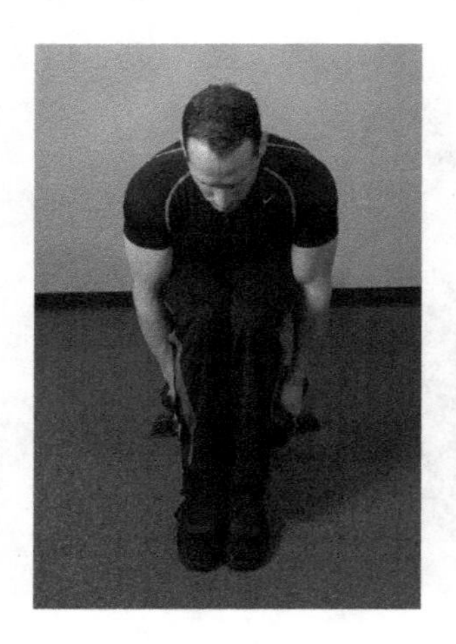

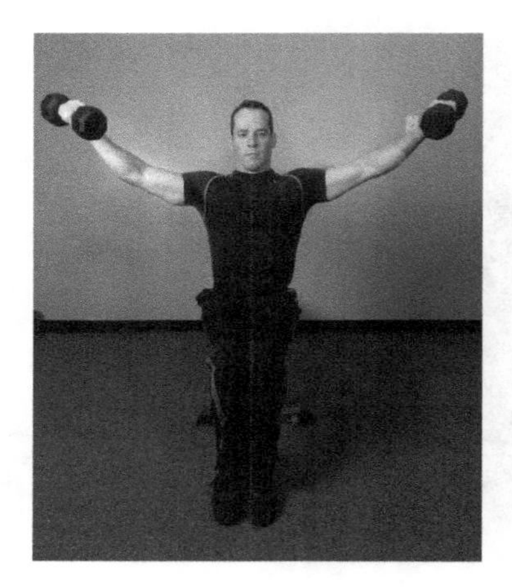

## Start

## Finish

Hinging from the hip keeping the back straight lean forward slightly. Touch the dumbells underneath your legs, looking down at a 45 degree angle past the knees. Now slowly move upright while at the same time raising the dumbells up just past shoulder height. Turn the thumbs down slightly. The pinkies will be higher. Keep back straight. Return slowly, coming back down into the starting position. Repeat the sequence until all repetitions are achieved. Rest, take 6 deep breaths, then continue your next set.

# Seated Bicep Curl

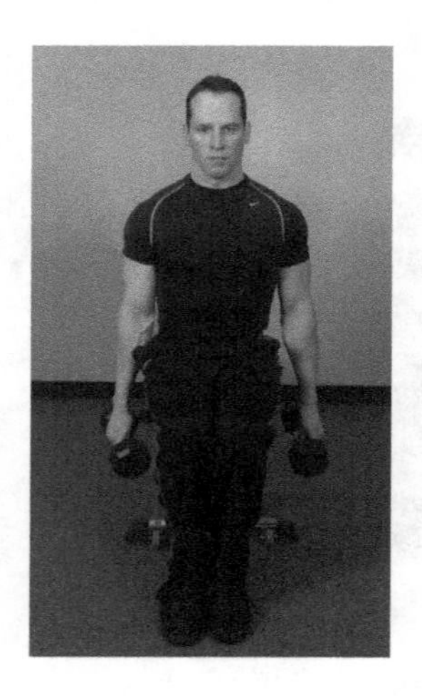

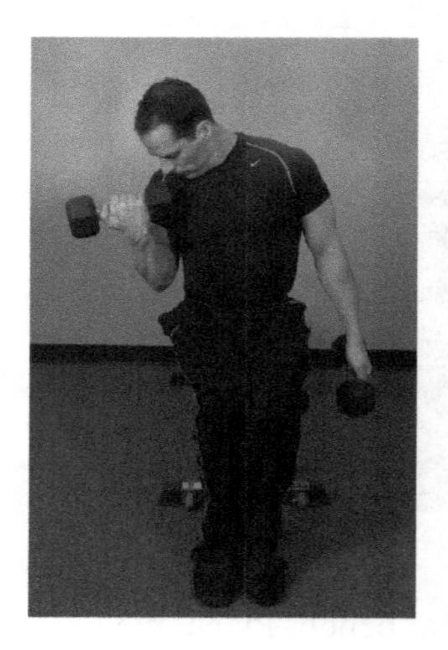

## Start

## Finish

Sitting in a chair or at the end of a flat bench keeping your back straight. Start with the dumbells down to your sides, arms extended. Now curl one dumbell up, turning and touching the bell to the shoulder. Look down at the bicep. Keep the elbow in tight to the body. Alternate arms.

# Tricep Kickback

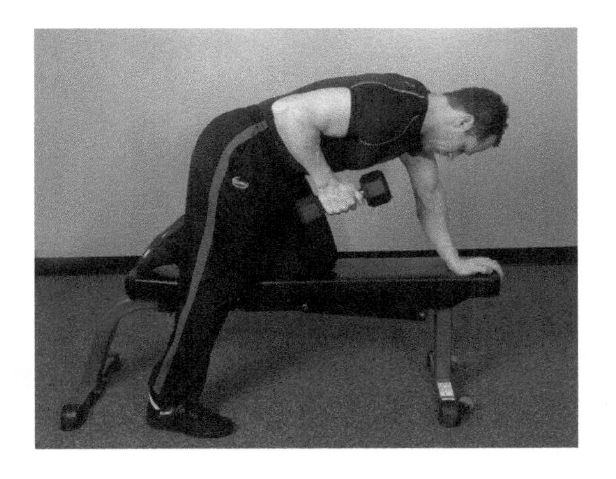

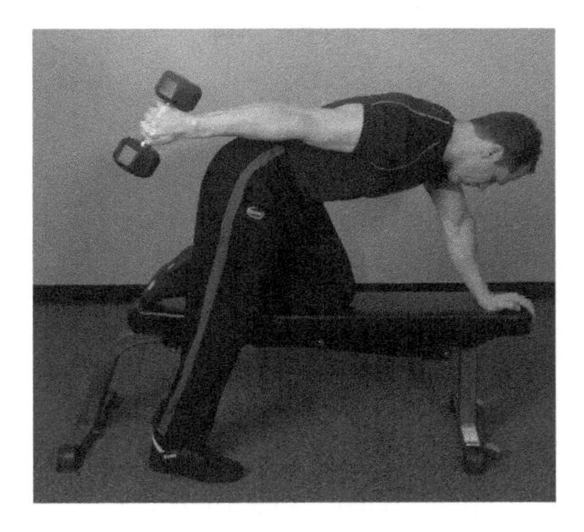

## Start

## Finish

Kneeling on a bench brace yourself with one hand placing it on the bench with arm extended. Now with the other arm keep the elbow high parallel to the floor. The dumbell remains at a 90 degree position at the start. Extend the arm, forcefully contracting the back of the arm (tricep). Hold contraction for a two second count. Return to starting position. Keep elbow up the entire time. Repeat sequence until all repetitions are achieved. Rest, take 6 deep breaths, then continue your next set.

# Frog Sit-Ups

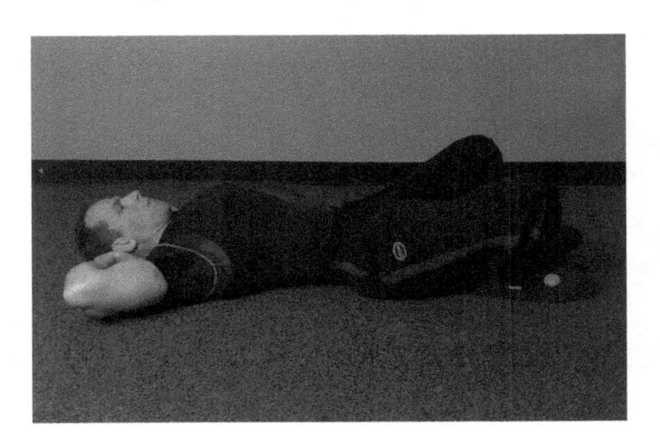

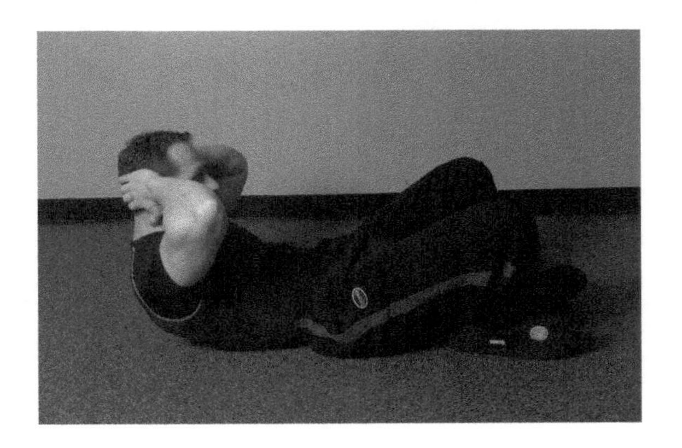

## Start

## Finish

Place your hands behind your head. Cross legs, keeping knees down toward floor. Exhale forcefully through pursed lips. Contract abdominals tightly. Blow all of the air out, fully contracting the abdominals. Avoid lifting knees up, keep them down. Return to starting position.

## Home Program:
# Program II:

- Dumbell Lunges
- Dumbell Chest Fly
- Bentover Row
- Upright Row
- Standing Bicep Curl
- Tricep Bench Dips
- Abdominal Bicycle

This program is designed for the home setting. All you need is a small dumbell set ranging from 5-12 pounds. When you become more advanced you may want to consider upgrading your dumbell set to 15-25 pounds. I suggest that you do Program I for two weeks then switch over to Program II. Changing programs every two weeks will keep your muscles from adapting to the exercises. It will help keep the muscles stimulated. Also, it helps keep you motivated.

# Dumbell Lunges

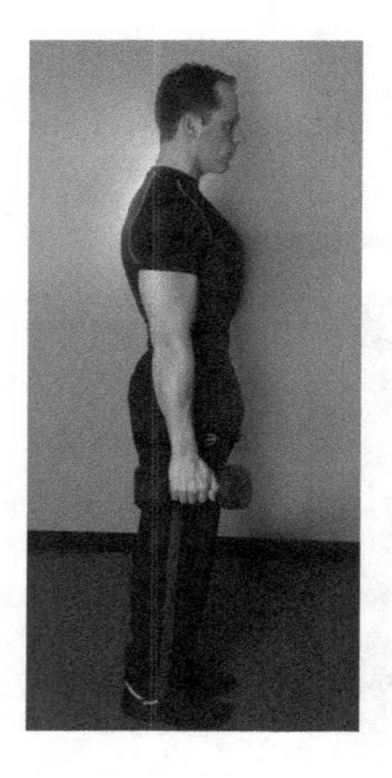

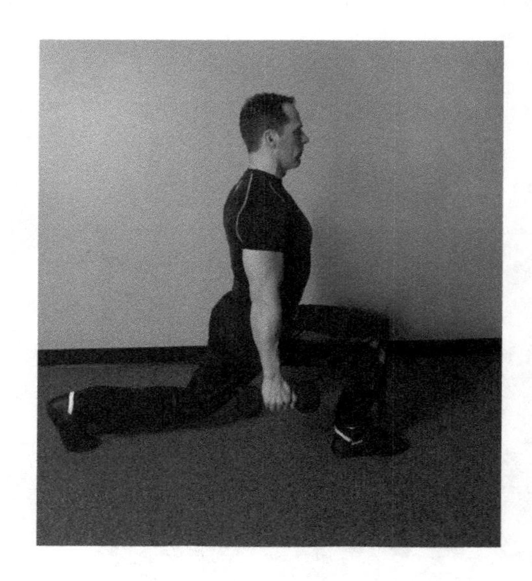

## Start

## Finish

Standing erect, with dumbells to the side of your body, back straight. Lunge one foot out, drop down so that the leg is at a 80-90 degree position. Keep chest up and back straight. Stand back up. Alternate legs. Repeat the sequence until all repetitions are achieved. Rest, take 6 deep breaths, then continue your next set.

# Dumbell Chest Fly

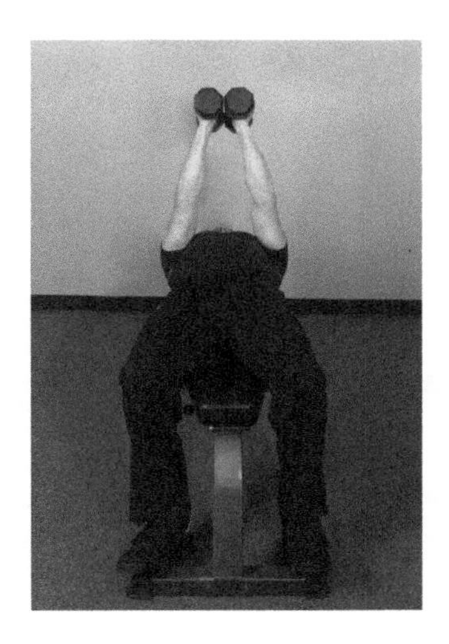

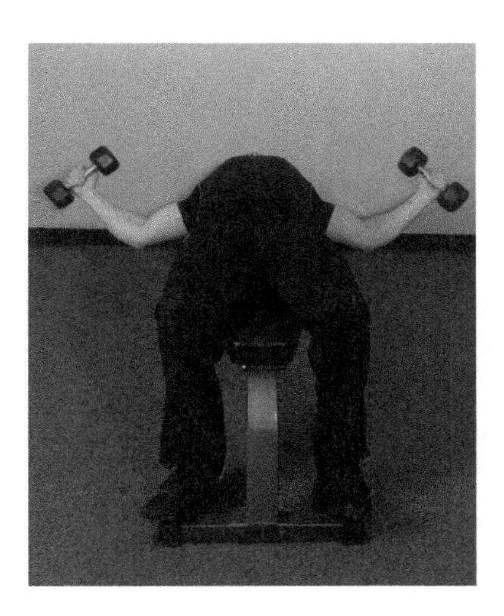

## Start

## Finish

Lie on a flat bench. Start with all four bells touching over your chest. Elbows slightly bent. Now bring the arms down in a wide pattern, keeping the elbows slightly bent. Stretch the chest completely by pulling elbows back slightly. Return to the starting position squeezing the chest tightly in the contracted position. Repeat the sequence until all repetitions are achieved. Rest, take 6 deep breaths, then continue your next set.

# Bentover Row

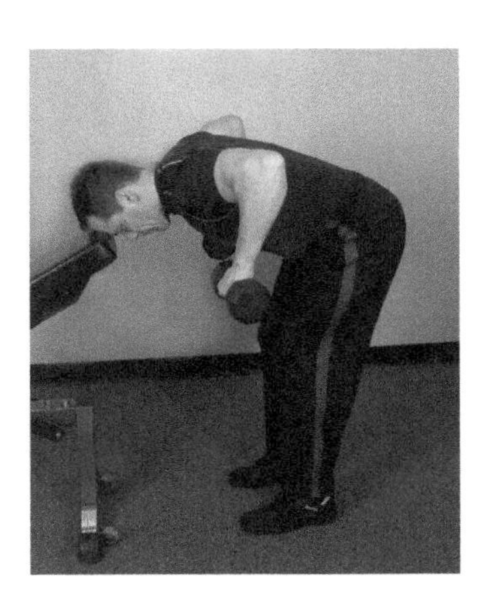

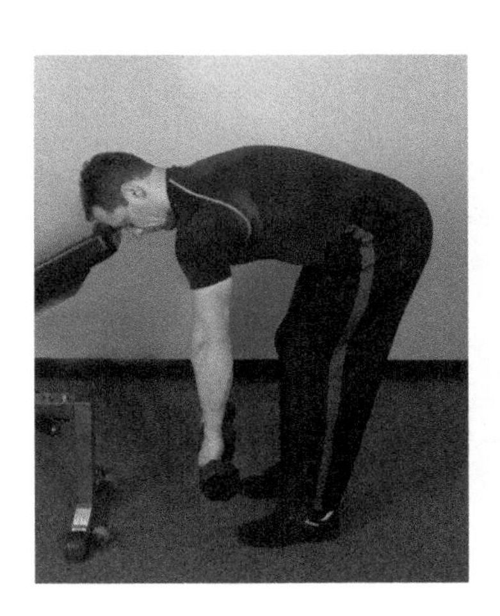

## Start

## Finish

Place head on a bench or table to support the back. With arms extended, pull dumbells up to the sides of the body. Keep elbows out wide, do not let them drop down toward the hips. Return slowly to the extended position. Repeat the sequence until all repetitions are achieved. Rest, take 6 deep breaths, then continue your next set.

# Upright Row

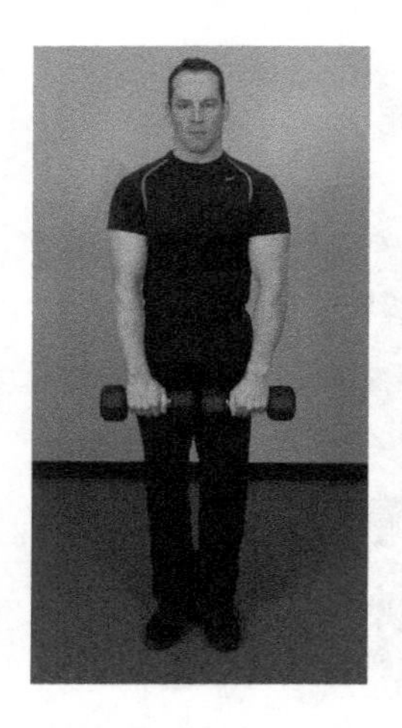

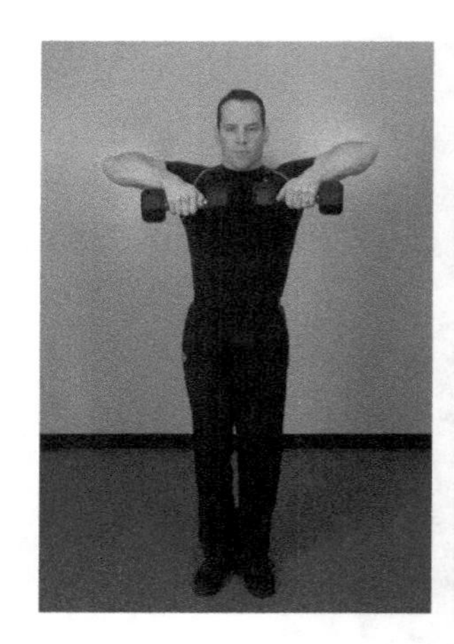

## Start Finish

Stand with your heels together and toes open, knees slightly bent. Keeping the chest up, pull the dumbells up elbows high. Lead with the elbows. Pull dumbells up level with the chest. Return slowly, keeping the back straight. Repeat the sequence until all repetitions are achieved. Rest, take 6 deep breaths, then continue your next set.

# Standing One Legged Bicep Curl

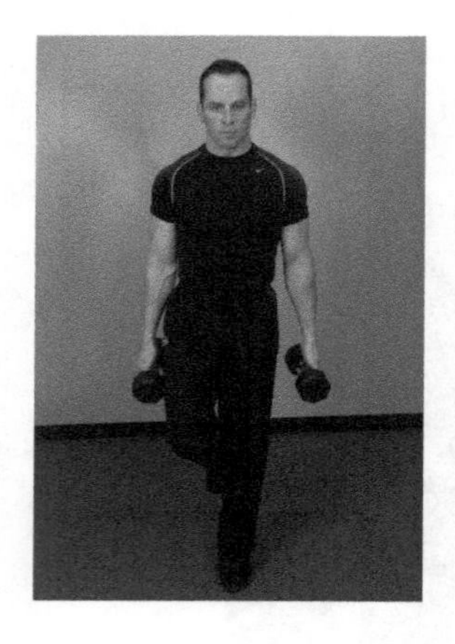

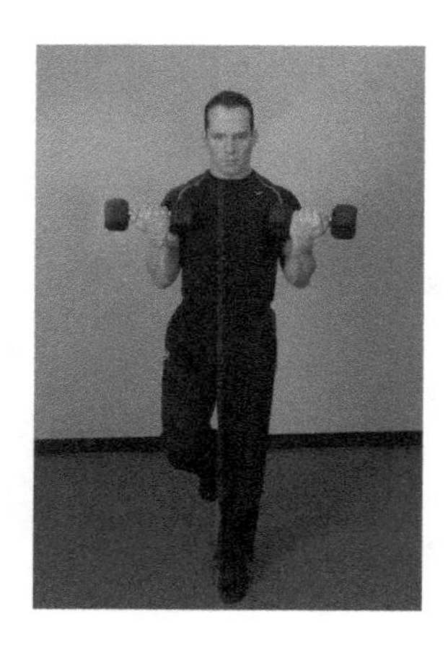

## Start Finish

Stand on one leg. Don't let the legs touch. Start with arms extended and dumbells next to the sides of the body. Curl the dumbells up toward the deltoids. Turn pinkies up slightly, keeping elbows down close to the body. Repeat the sequence on other leg. Rest, take 6 deep breaths, then continue your next set.

# Tricep Bench Dips

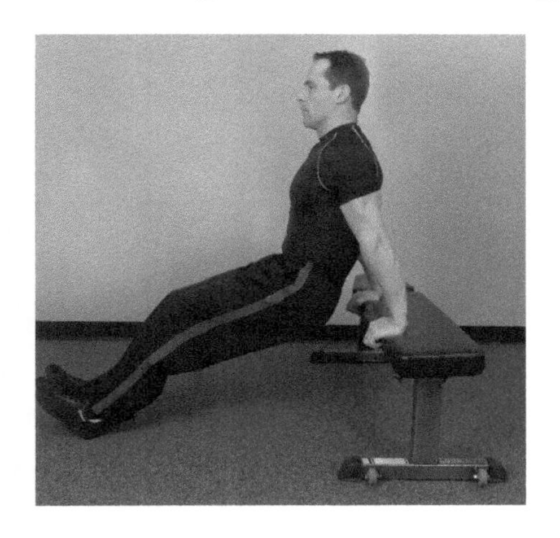

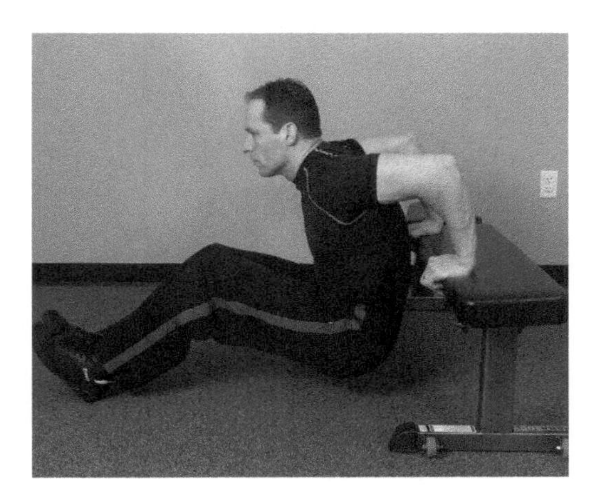

## Start

## Finish

Starting with hands holding onto the side of a bench or chair, shuffle off the bench so your bottom is off suspended.. Your arms are extended supporting your weight. Stay on your heels. Now dip down toward the floor stretching the chest and shoulders. The arm should get into a 90 degree position to be effective. Now push up returning into the extended position. This is a challenging exercise. If you cannot perform it go back to doing the tricep kickback.

# Abdominal Bicycle

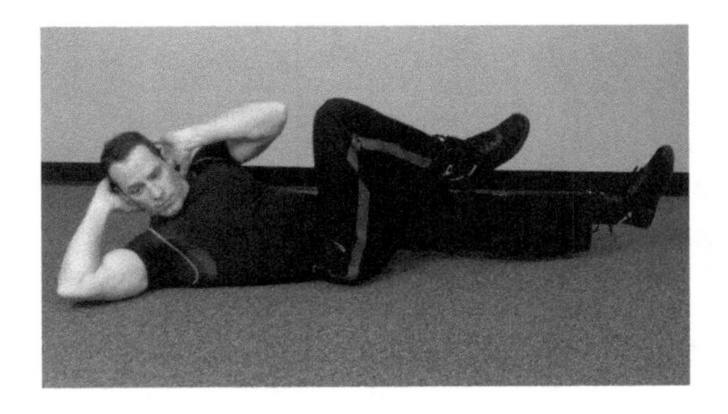

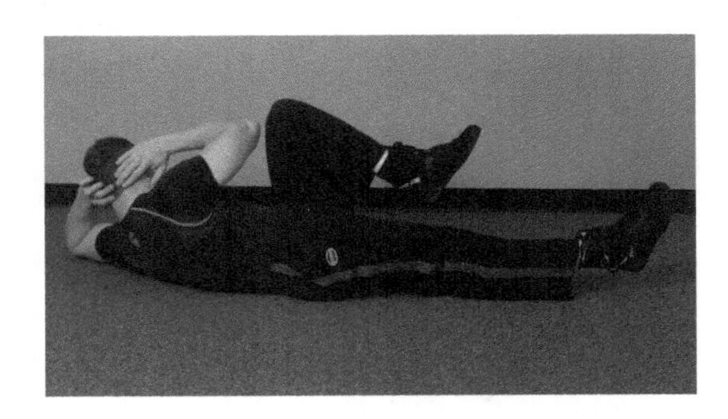

## Start

## Finish

Lying on the floor, hands behind head. Draw one leg in toward the chest, keeping the other leg straight. Turn and rotate torso toward the knee that is drawn in. Now smoothly turn and rotate toward the other knee as you transfer legs. Move in a synchronized fashion, shoulder to knee, extending legs one at a time. Exhale turning to one side, inhale returning.

# In The Gym: General Conditioning

***Machine Program***

- Leg Press
- Seated Hamstring Curl
- Chest Press
- Back Row
- Lat Pulldown
- Shoulder Press
- Cable Bicep Curl
- Tricep Pressdown
- Ab Bench

This program is designed for the gym setting. The machines that I used for this program a typically found in most gyms. If the machine is not available to you ask the fitness professional at the gym to help you choose a similar exercise. When working with machines, it is important to go slow. Do not let the weights bang. You want to perform a smooth, consistent motion.

## Leg Press

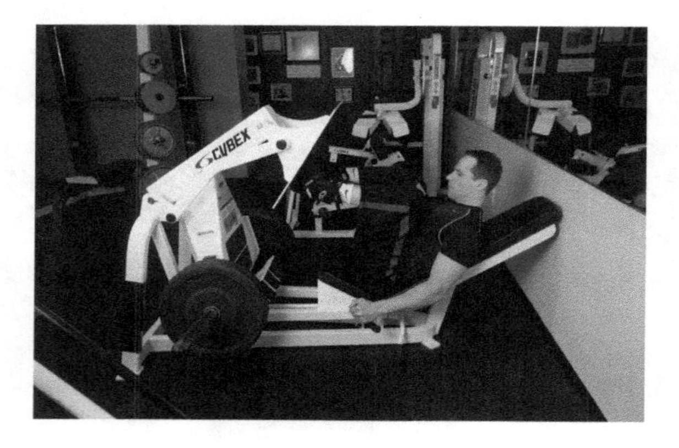


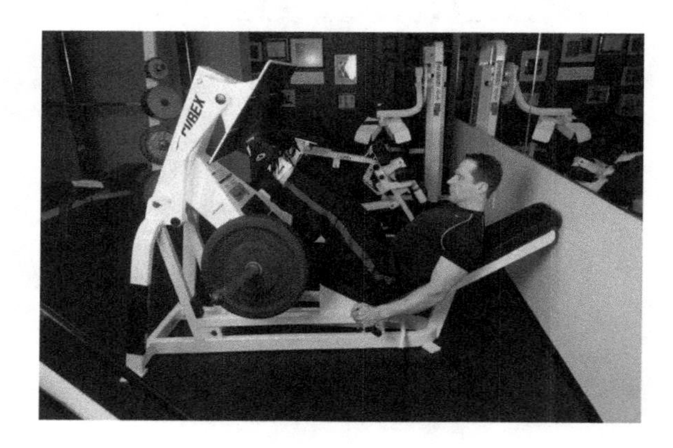

**Start** **Finish**

Start with feet shoulder width apart, toes slightly turned open. Keep back down, pressed firmly against seat. Bend the knees bringing down the sled. Come down only far enough so that the back doesn't come off the seat. Now push sled back up extending the legs. Repeat sequence until all repetitions are achieved. Rest, take 6 deep breaths, then continue your next set.

# Seated Hamstring Curl

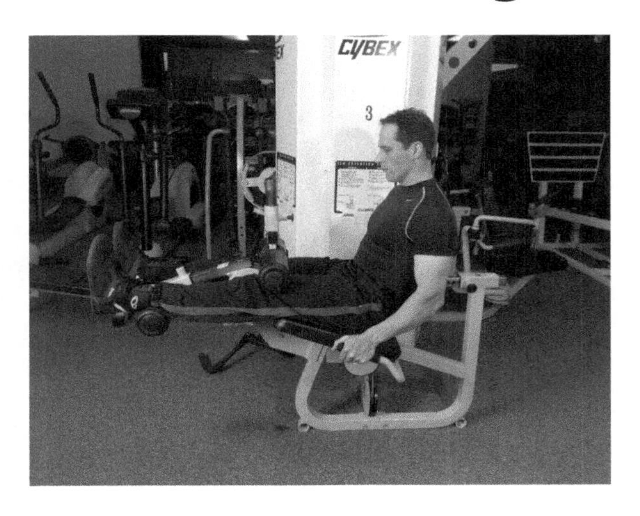


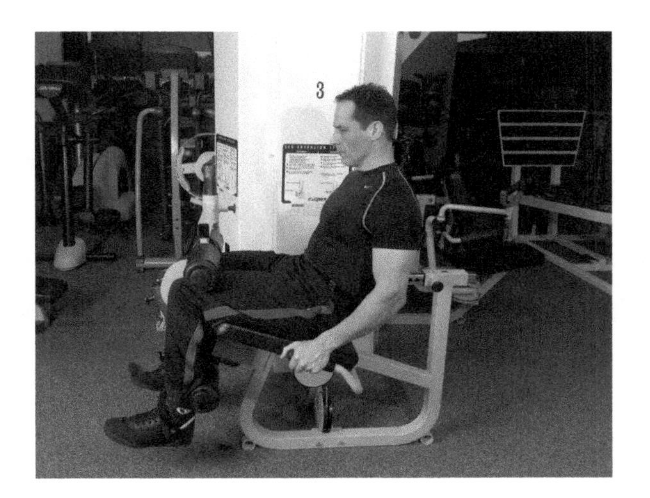


## Start Finish

Start with your legs in an extended position. Keep back firmly pressed against seat. Curl the legs down to a 90 degree angle. Avoid arching the back. Keep the abdominals tight. Repeat sequence until all repetitions are achieved. Rest, take 6 deep breaths, then continue your next set.

# Chest Press

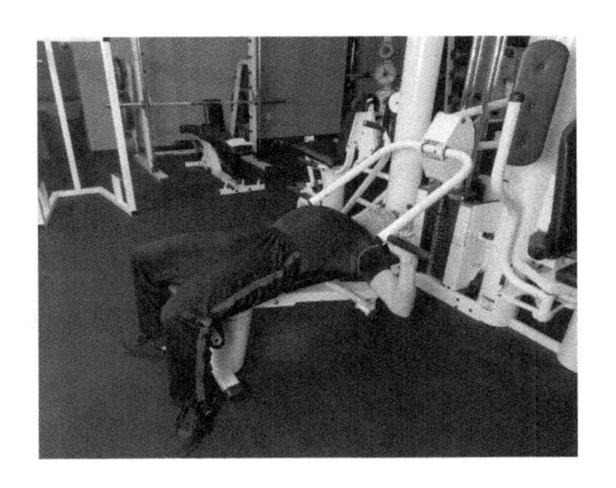

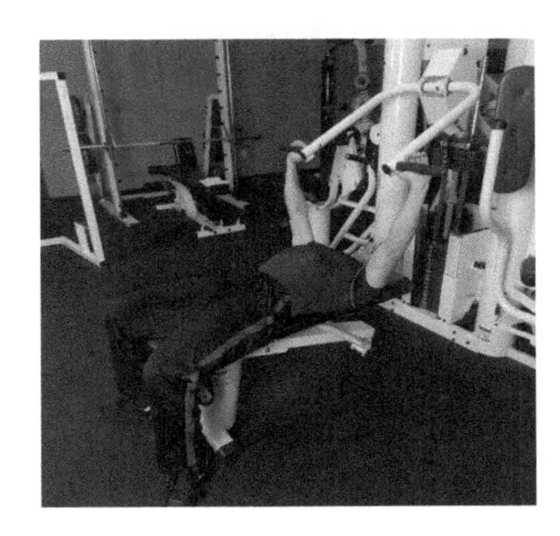

## Start Finish

Lie down. Keep the elbows wide to stretch the chest. Exhale and push the bar up. Avoid extending the arms completely, keep a slight bend in the elbows. Return slowly, avoid banging the weights. Repeat the sequence until all repetitions are achieved. Rest, take 6 deep breaths, then continue your next set.

# Seated Back Row

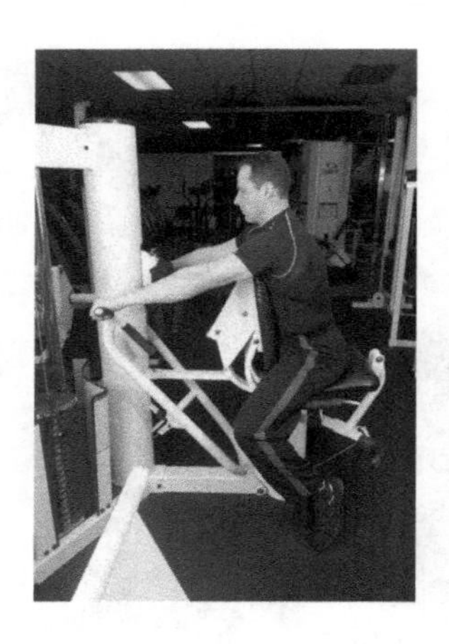

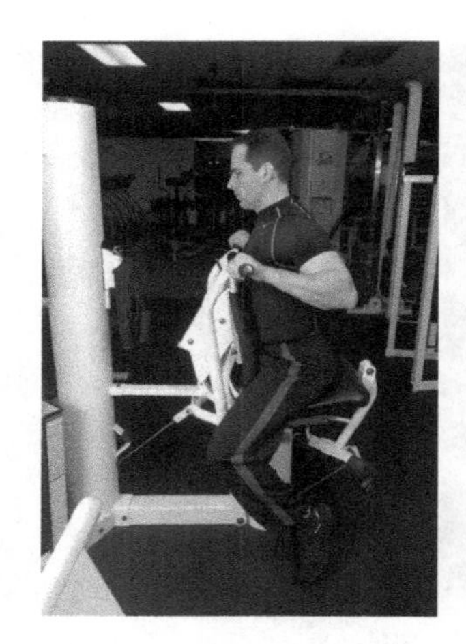

**Start** **Finish**

Grab the handles with arms extended. Keeping the back straight, pull the bar toward the body keeping the chest in contact with the pad. Contract the back tightly. Hold contraction for 1-2 seconds. Release and return slowly to the starting position. Repeat the sequence until all repetitions are achieved. Rest, take 6 deep breaths, then continue your next set.

# Lat Pulldown

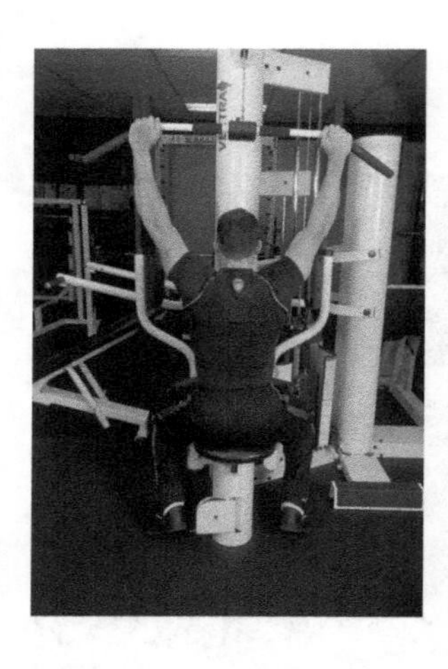

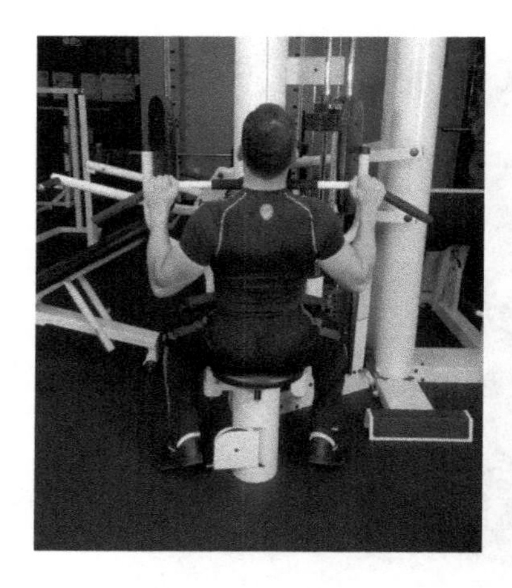

**Start** **Finish**

Sit under the lat bar. Grab the bar a little more than shoulder width. Pull bar down keeping the chest up. Bring bar down toward the front of the body. Contract the back tightly. Drive elbows down toward the sides of the body. Hold contraction for 1-2 seconds. Return slowly. Repeat the sequence until all repetitions are achieved. Rest, take 6 deep breaths, then continue your next set.

# Shoulder Press

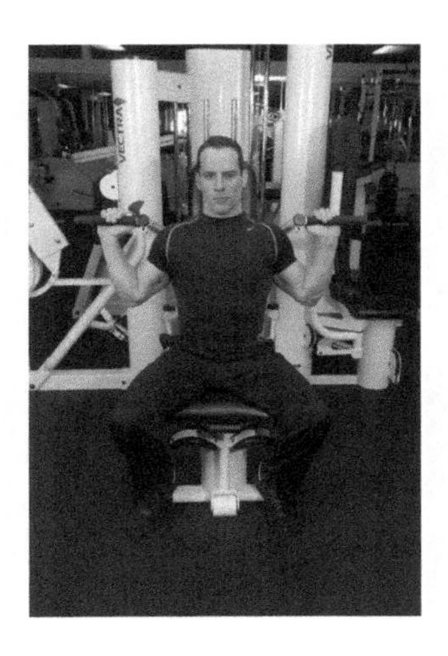

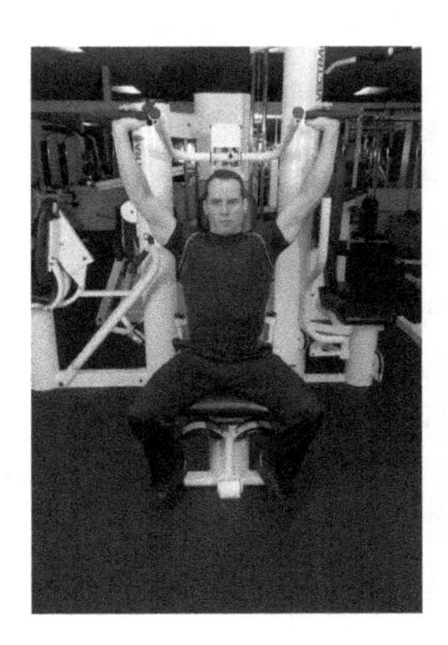

## Start

## Finish

Start by sitting upright holding onto the bar, elbows down toward sides. Press bar up. Avoid extending the arms fully. Keep the elbows slightly bent. Return slowly, avoid banging weights. Repeat the sequence until all repetitions are achieved. Rest, take 6 deep breaths, then continue your next set.

# Cable Bicep Curl

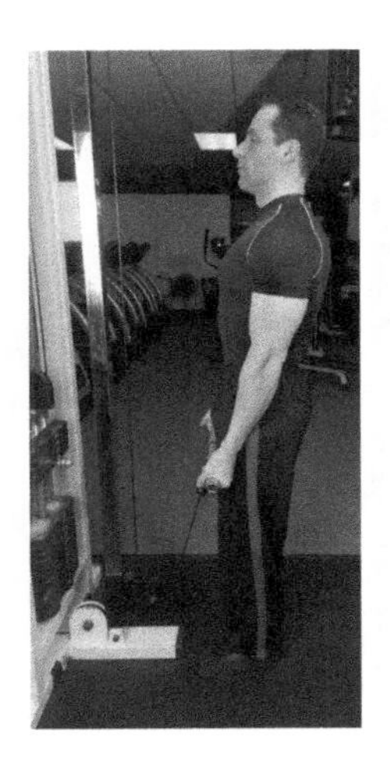

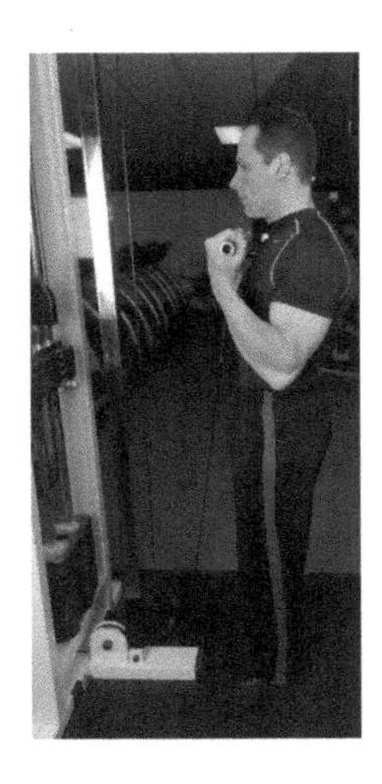

## Start

## Finish

Stand erect, chest up, arms extended, elbows down and close to the body. Curl bar up toward shoulders. Contract biceps tightly. Keep elbows down throughout entire exercise. Return slowly, avoid banging weights. Repeat the sequence until all repetitions are achieved. Rest, take 6 deep breaths, then continue your next set.

# Tricep Pressdown

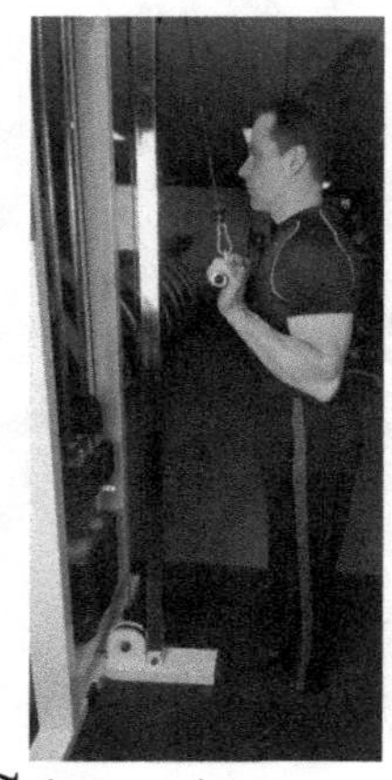

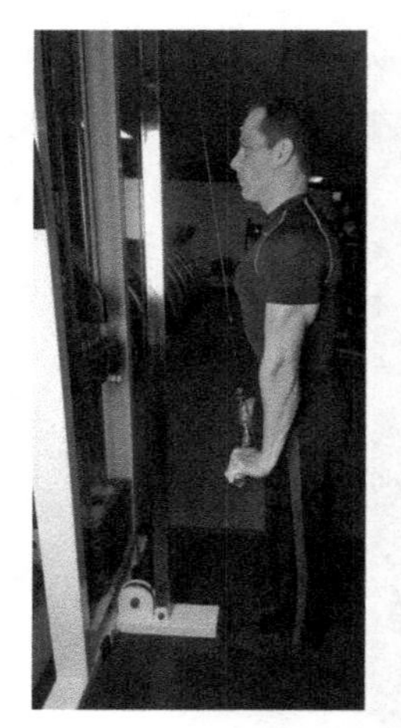

**Start** **Finish**

Grab the bar, keeping it close to the chest. Keep elbows down next to the sides of the body. Pull the bar down extending arms completely, contracting the triceps fully. Hold contraction and return slowly, keeping elbows close to the body. Return slowly, avoid banging weights. Repeat sequence until all repetitions are achieved. Rest, take 6 deep breaths, then continue your next set.

# Ab Bench

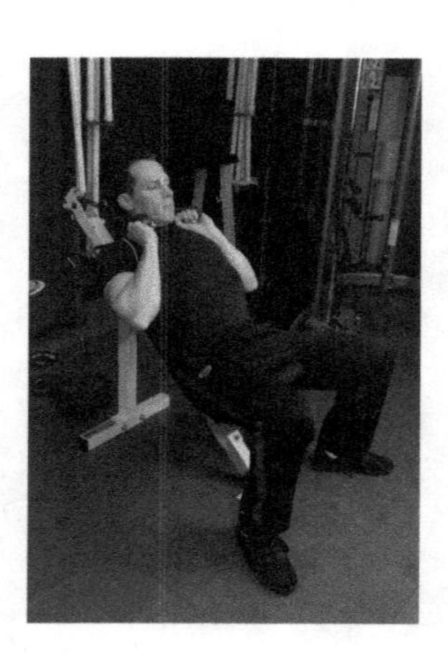

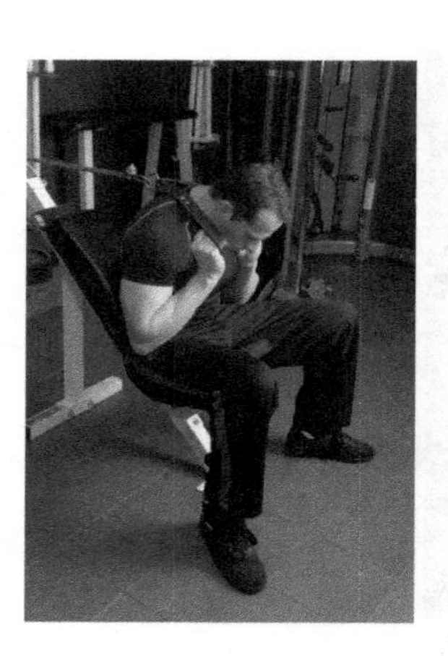

**Start** **Finish**

Grab handles. Keep handles close to the chest. Draw abdominals in. Flex forward blowing the air out of the abdominals. Contract the abdominals tightly. Release and return. Inhale completely on the way back. Repeat the sequence until all repetitions are achieved. Rest, take 6 deep breaths, then continue your next set.

# In The Gym: General Conditioning

***Free Weight Program***

- Barbell Squat
- Ball Hamstring Tuck
- Dumbell Flat Bench Chest Press
- Lat Pulldown
- Bent Over Dumbell Row (Head on Bench)
- Seated Lateral Raise
- Barbell Bicep Curl
- Tricep DB Overhead Extension
- Abdominal Forearm Plank
- Abdominal Side Arm Plank

# Barbell Squat

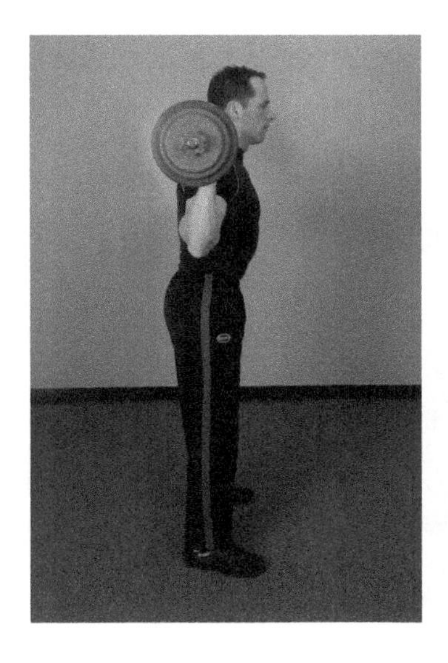

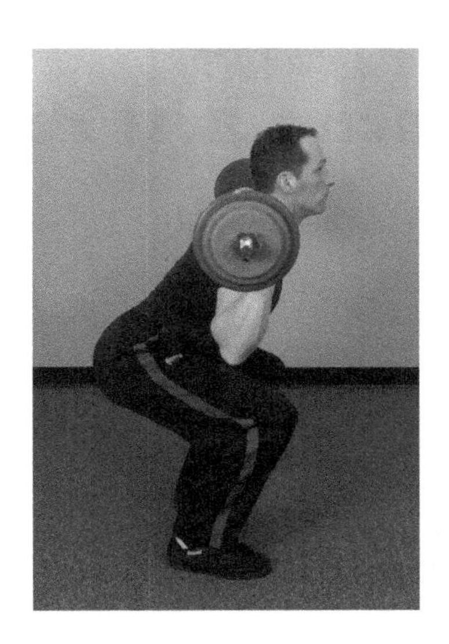

# Start Finish

Start with the bar on the back between the shoulders. Press up on the bar to relieve pressure on the vertebras. Open up your stance, toes slightly turned open. Hinge from the hip, keeping the back straight squat down to 80-90 degree knee flexion. Hold for 1-2 seconds. Push up through the legs standing back up, keeping heels firmly pressed on the floor. Tuck hips forward when coming back into the erect position. Repeat the sequence until all repetitions are achieved. Rest, take 6 deep breaths, then continue your next set.

# Ball Hamstring Tuck

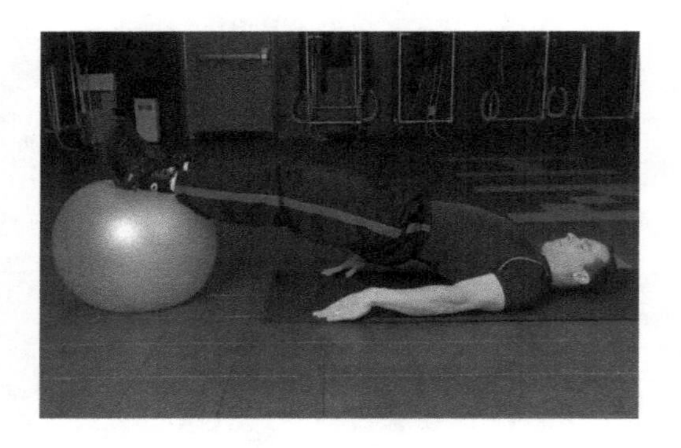

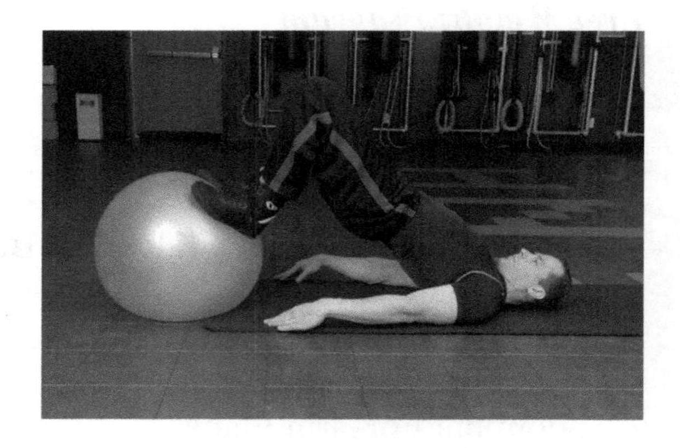

## Start Finish

Lying down, place feet on a therapy ball. Lift the hips up off the floor. Support yourself by keeping your arms extended on the floor. Pull the ball in toward you, keeping the hips up. Return straightening the legs back to the starting position. Keep hips up off the floor the entire time. Repeat the sequence until all repetitions are achieved. Rest, take 6 deep breaths, then continue your next set.

# Dumbell Flat Bench Chest Press

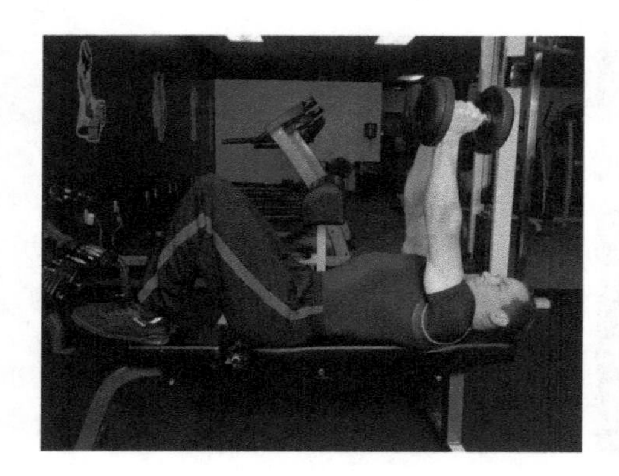

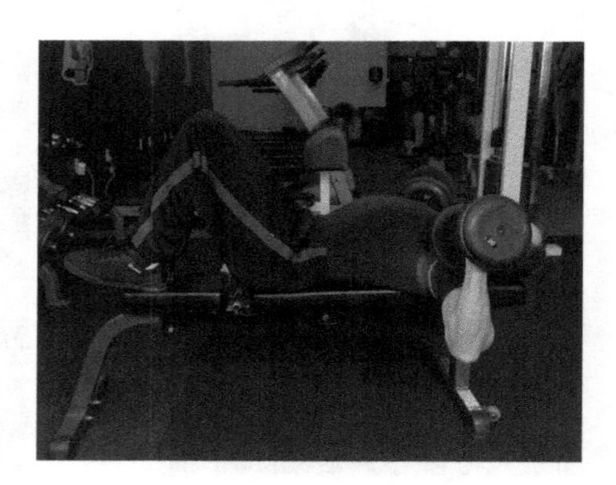

## Start Finish

Start with all four bells touching above your chest, elbows slightly bent. Bring the dumbells down flaring out your elbows wide to stretch the chest. The dumbells end up spread out with the palms facing the feet. Press weight back up, slowly turning the hands in as you ascend to the starting position. Tightly contract the chest for a 1-2 second count. Repeat the sequence until all repetitions are achieved. Rest, take 6 deep breaths, then continue your next set.

# Lat Pulldown

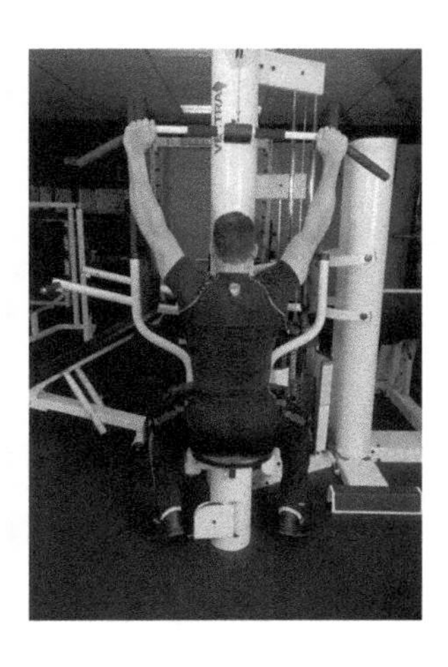

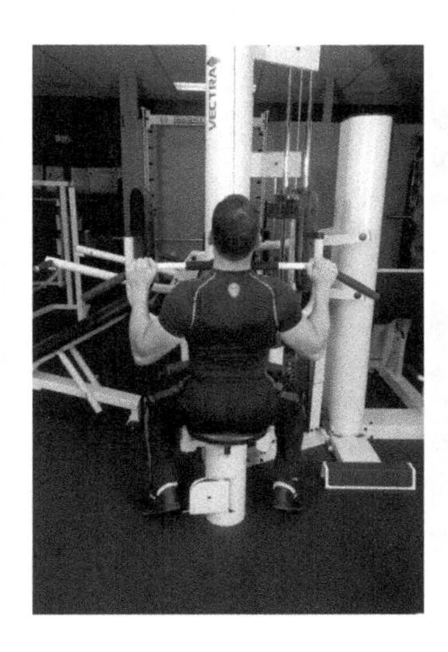

## Start

## Finish

Sit under the lat bar. Grab the bar a little more than shoulder width. Pull bar down keeping the chest up. Bring bar down toward the front of the body. Contract the back tightly. Drive elbows down toward the sides of the body. Hold contraction for 1-2 seconds. Return slowly. Repeat the sequence until all repetitions are achieved. Rest, take 6 deep breaths, then continue your next set.

# Bent Over Dumbell Row (Head on Bench)

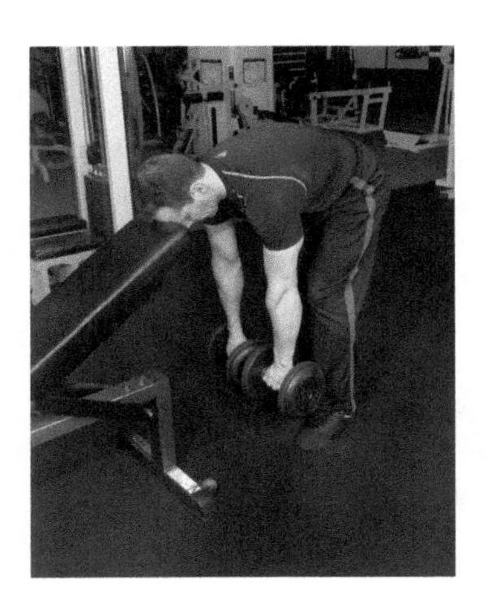

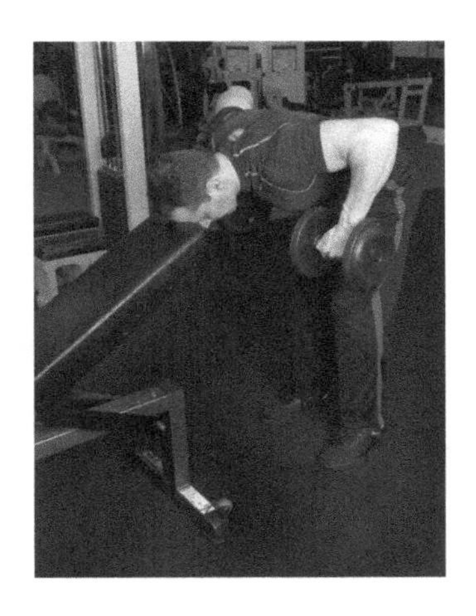

## Start

## Finish

Place head on a bench or table to support the back. With arms extended, pull dumbells up to the sides of the body. Keep elbows out wide, do not let them drop down toward the hips. Return slowly to extended position. Repeat the sequence until all repetitions are achieved. Rest, take 6 deep breaths, then continue your next set.

# Seated Lateral Raise

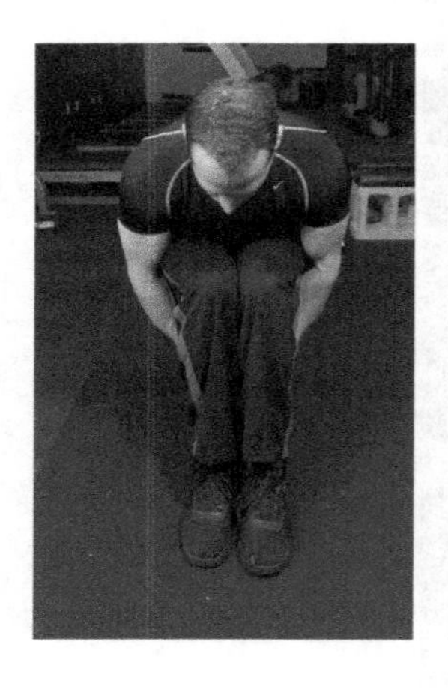

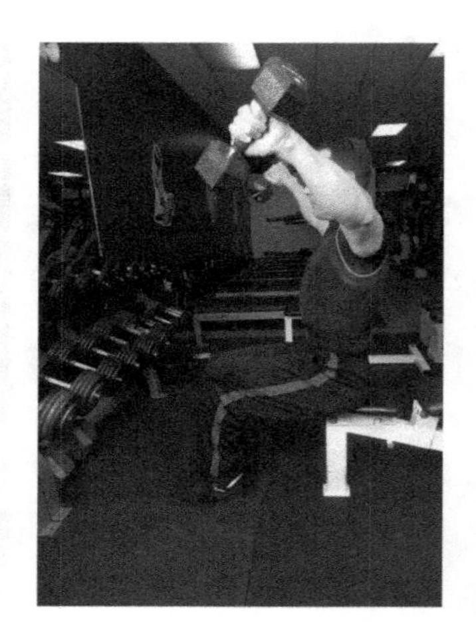

## Start

## Finish

Hinging from the hip, keep the back straight and lean forward slightly. Touch the dumbells underneath your legs, looking down at a 45 degree angle past the knees. Now slowly move upright while at the same time raising the dumbells up just past shoulder height. Turn the thumbs down slightly. The pinkies will be higher. Keep back straight. Return slowly, coming back down into the starting position. Repeat the sequence until all repetitions are achieved. Rest, take 6 deep breaths, then continue your next set.

# Barbell Bicep Curl

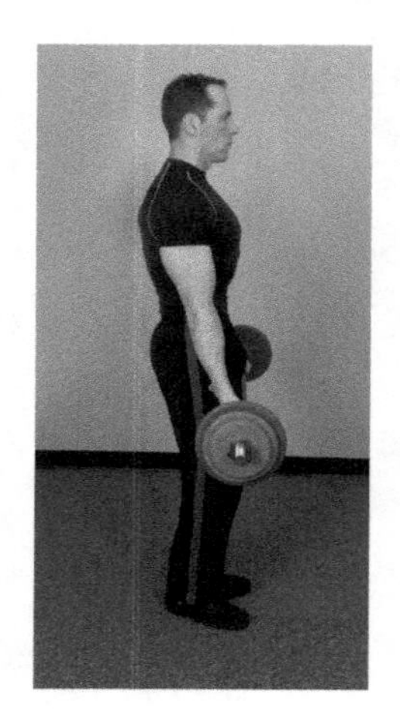

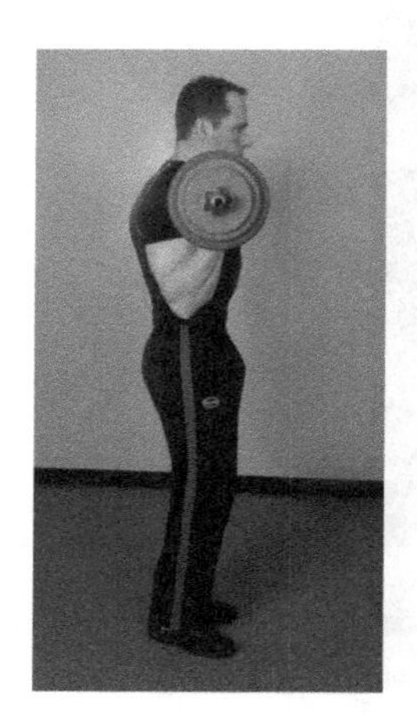

## Start

## Finish

Standing erect. Heels together, toes turned out, knees slightly bent. Start with barbell on thighs with arms extended. Keep elbows pressed close to the sides of the body. Curl the bar up tight to the shoulders. Hold contraction for 1-2 seconds. Don't swing weight up. Return slowly.

# Tricep Dumbell Overhead Extension

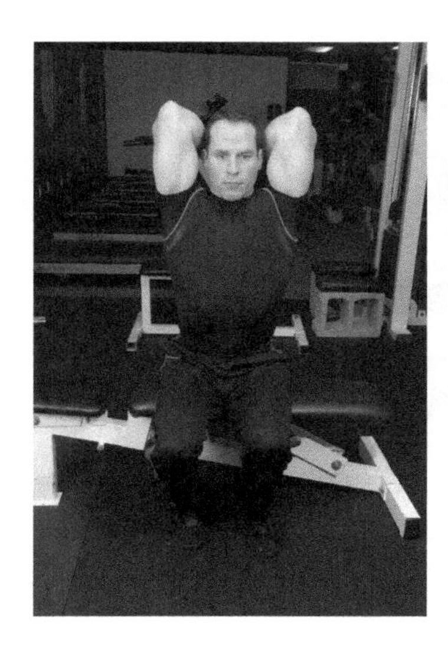
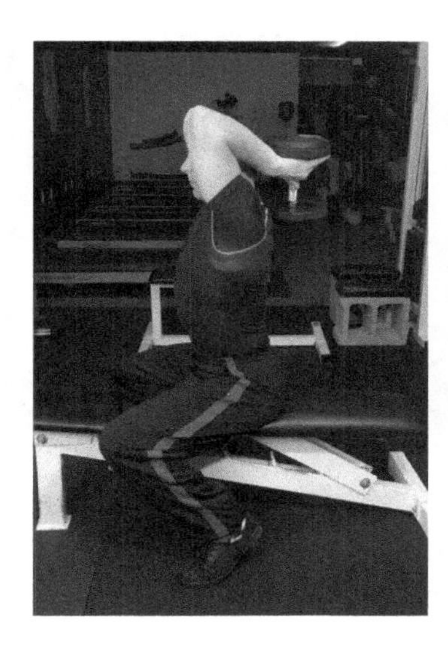
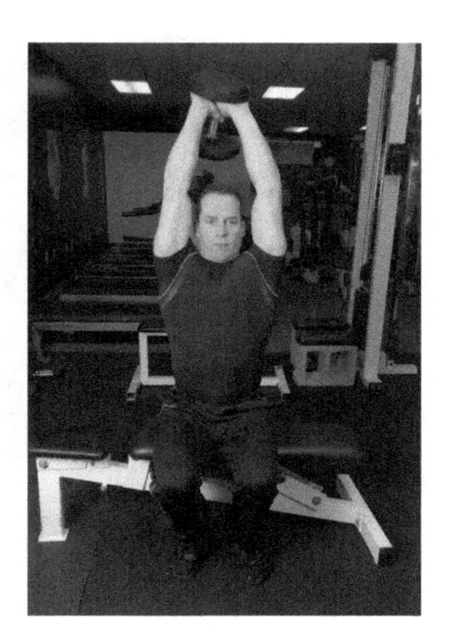

## Start Finish

Sitting on a bench hold a dumbell with both hands cupping the bell. Keep elbows close to the head, pointing up toward the ceiling. Stretch the triceps by allowing the dumbell to drop down behind your head. Now extend the arms overhead, squeezing the triceps forcefully into contraction. Hold for 1-2 seconds then return to starting position. Keep elbows up and close to the head throughout the entire motion. Repeat the sequence until all repetitions are achieved. Rest, take 6 deep breaths, then continue your next set.

# Abdominal Forearm Plank

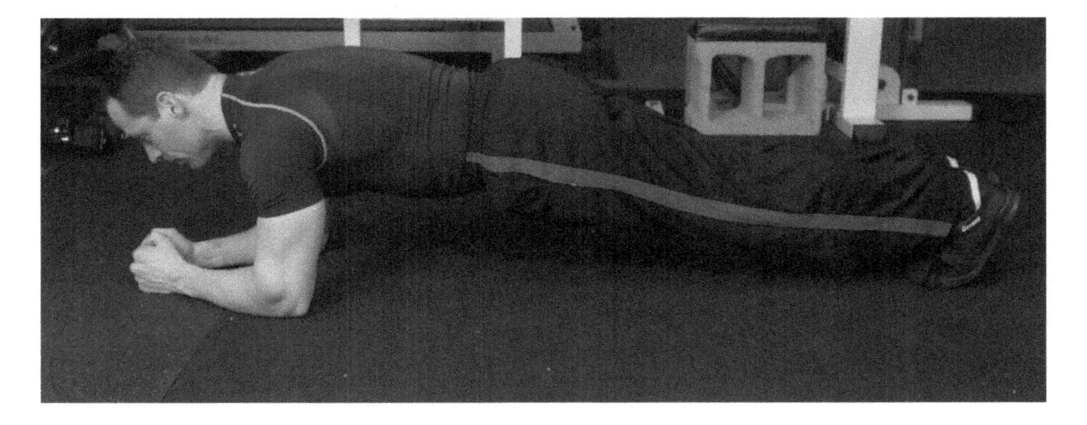

Hold yourself up on your toes and forearms. Keep the spine neutral by keeping the hips up in line with the ankle, knee, hip and shoulder joint. Avoid arching back. Avoid dropping the shoulder blades down producing faulty form. Keep the back straight. Contract the abdominals tightly to support the lower back. A set consists of holding this formation for 30- 60 seconds.

# Abdominal Side Arm Plank

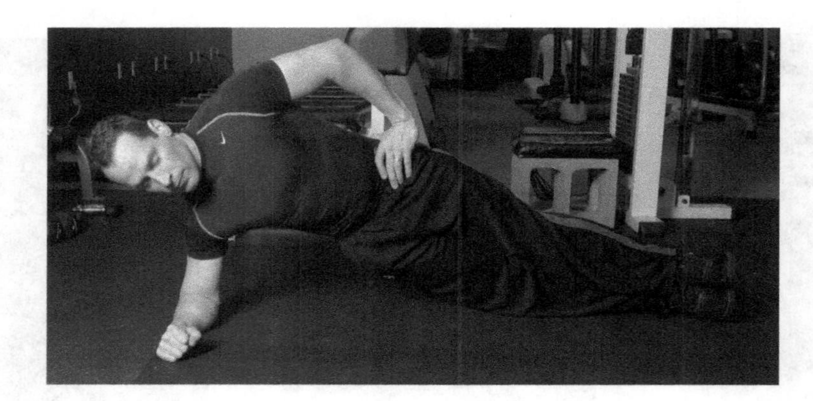

Hold yourself up on your forearm perpendicular to the body and the side of your foot. The other hand is on the hip. Keeping the hips up off the floor. The spine needs to stay straight. Close your eyes to make this posture harder. A set consists of holding this formation for 30- 60 seconds.

# In The Gym: Bone Building Emphasis

***Beginner***
• Barbell Squat
• Deadlift
• Flat Bench Barbell Chest Press

This program is designed to help increase overall body density. These three exercises work the entire skeletal system. To build bone there must be enough stimulation to force the bone to bend. The bending allows osteoblasts to migrate and help build more bone. Form is critical on these exercises so take heed. These exercises can be done at home but are more suitable in a gym setting. In a gym a professional fitness instructor can watch your form to make sure you are doing them correctly.

# Barbell Squat

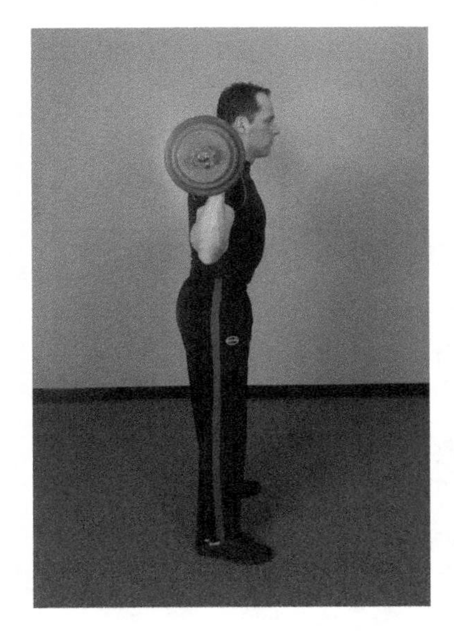

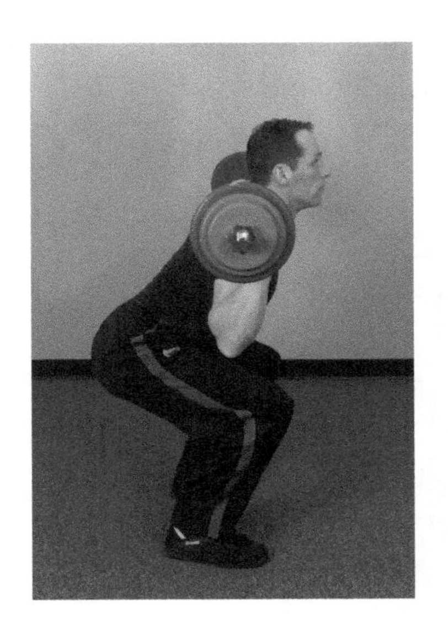

## Start

## Finish

Start with the bar on the back between the shoulders. Press up on the bar to relieve pressure on the vertebras. Open up your stance, toes slightly turned open. Hinge from the hip, keeping the back straight squat down to 80-90 degree knee flexion. Hold for 1-2 seconds. Push up through the legs standing back up, keeping heels firmly pressed on the floor. Tuck hips forward when coming back into the erect position. Repeat the sequence until all repetitions are achieved. Rest, take 6 deep breaths, then continue your next set.

# Deadlift

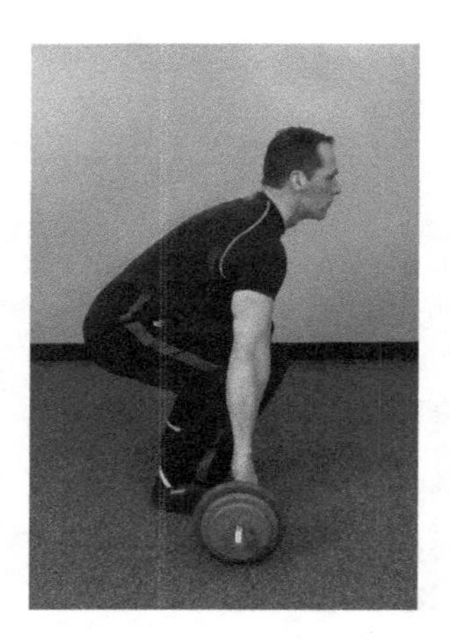

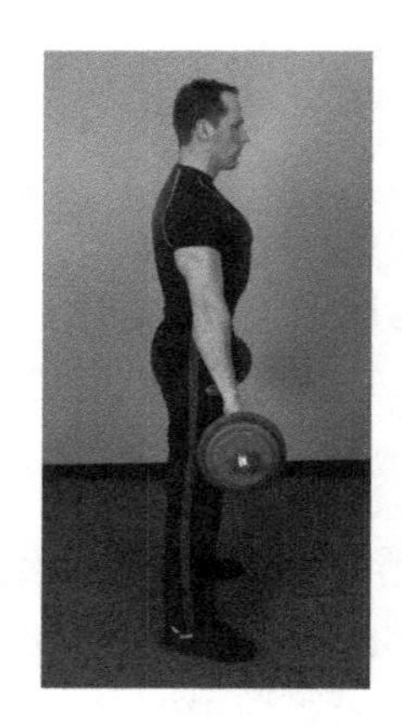

**Start** **Finish**

Start with your feet shoulder width, toes slightly opened up. Squat down, grabbing the bar a little more than shoulder width apart , knees flexed at 80-90 degrees. Look straight ahead, chest up, hips hinged, bottom down. Stand up clearing the bar over the knees. Straighten the hips and knees into extension at the same time. Timing is important here. When done correctly the chest will be high, glutes tight, hips tucked in, abdominals drawn in. Return, hinging at the hip and bringing the bar back onto the floor

# Dumbell Flat Bench Chest Press

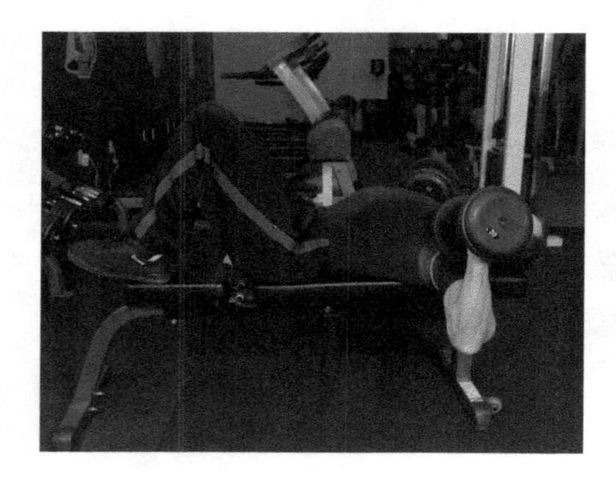

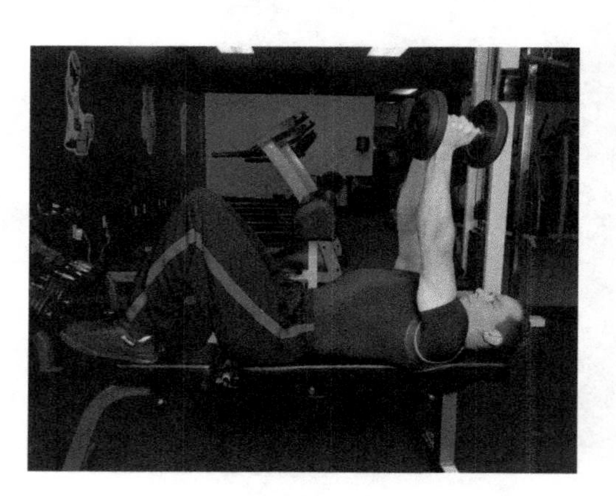

**Start** **Finish**

Start with all four bells touching above your chest. Elbows slightly bent. Bring the dumbells down flaring our your elbows wide to stretch the chest. The dumbells end up spread out with the palms facing the feet. Press weight back up slowly turning the hands in as you ascend to the starting position. Tightly contract the chest for a 1-2 second count. Repeat the sequence until all repetitions are achieved. Rest, take 6 deep breaths, then continue your next set.

# Functional Training Program

***Beginner***

- Clean and Press
- One Arm Single Leg Cable Pull
- Wood Chop
- Transverse Cable Rotation
- Walking Lunges
- Lateral Strides w/Dumbell Press

***Advanced***

- Clean and Press
- One Arm Single Leg Cable Pull
- Wood Chop
- Transverse Cable Rotation
- Walking Lunges
- Lateral Strides w/Dumbell Press
- Deadlift
- Medicine Ball Push Ups
- Medicine Ball Up Wood Chop

Functional training is defined as performing exercises that simulate functions of human movement. The theory is that the body moves and operates in three planes of motion multi-plane (frontal, sagittal, transverse) and that all human movement is synergistic and uses multi-joint operation to achieve a task. For example lifting a bag of groceries from your car requires the use of legs, back, core control, and arms to achieve the task. So, by doing exercises that mimic the same movements as what a body would do during work, sports, or everyday activities then the body responds better to unstable and unpredictable environments. In addition, functional training is another way of challenging the muscles and nervous system by providing a greater fat burning effect while activating more muscle. Perform 1-3 sets

# Clean and Press

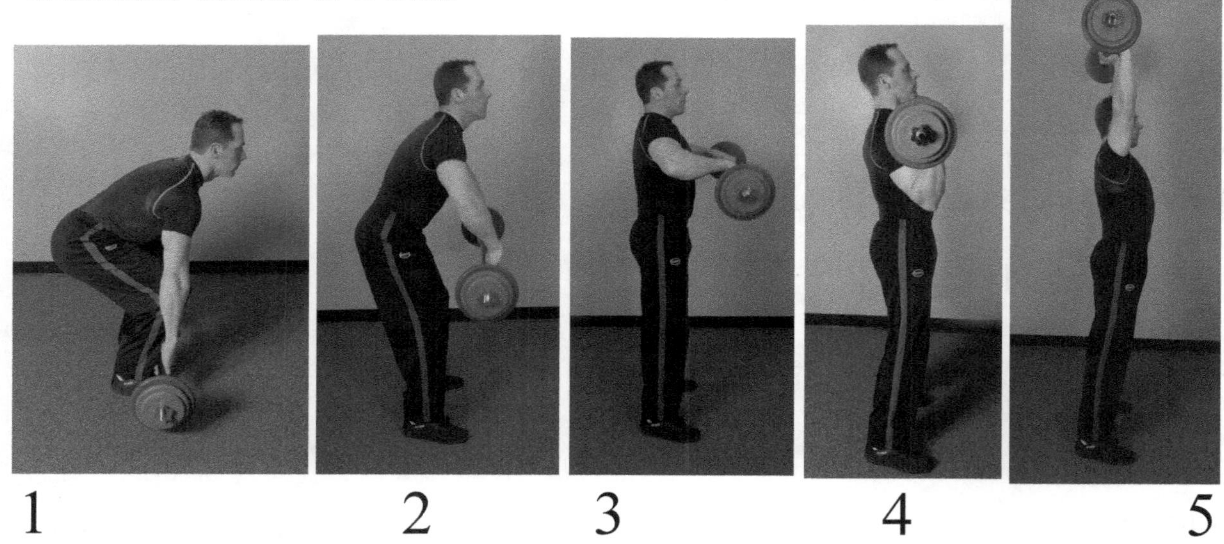


1. Start with your feet shoulder width, toes slightly opened up. Squat down, grabbing the bar a little more than shoulder width, knees flexed at 80-90 degrees. Look straight ahead, chest up, hips hinged, bottom down.

2. Begin standing up. Keep hips low, chest comes up. With momentum, swing the bar out in front of your body. Keeping back neutral (no flexion).

3. Momentum will help the bar come up. You must move quickly to allow the bar to get up and to avoid using only shoulders to get the weight up. Essentially you are hoisting the bar up and catching it.

4. Catch the weight up onto the front of the chest. At this point you should be standing up erect. Tuck the hips forward to protect the lower back.

5. Now press the weight up over you head. Keep a wide stance to support the back. Avoid arching the back when the bar is over head.

* This is a great exercise. However, this is an advanced exercise and should be done in good form. If you have difficulty with this exercise I suggest you seek help from a professional fitness instructor to show you the exact movement.

# One Arm Single Leg Cable Pull

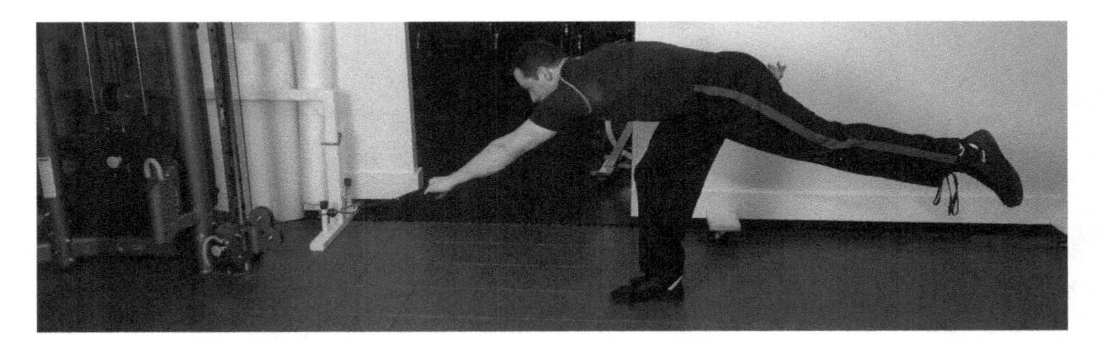

## Start

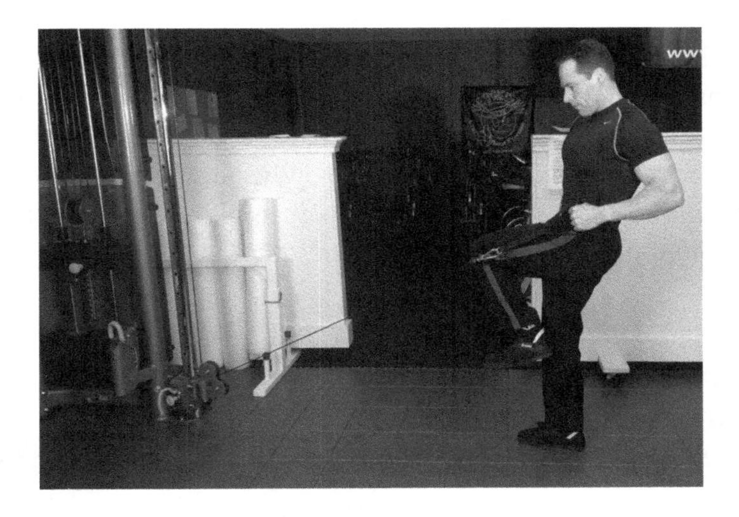

## Finish

Set up a low cable pulley with the handle attachment. Stand on one leg, with the other leg extended up off the ground. Keep the leg as straight as possible in line with the spin. Keep the back neutral (straight). Reach out with one hand extended holding onto the handle. The other arm is down and to the side of the body. Now slowly, and in a synchronized fashion pull the handle toward your body while standing upright with the leg coming toward the front of the body. Hip and knee flexion is 90 degrees at the completion of the pull. Your hand should be tight and close to the hip. This movement is a dynamic movement that requires balance and coordination. Your core strength will be challenged. Many muscles are working at one time to produce a single task. Focus on good form and work slowly until you get the hang of it. Then you can challenge yourself by going a little faster with good control.

# Wood Chop

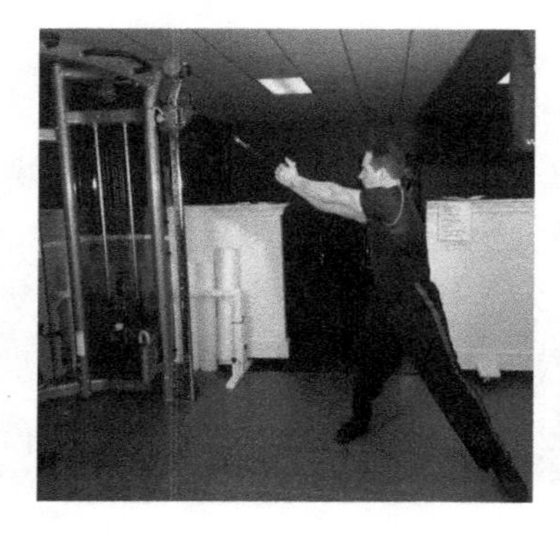

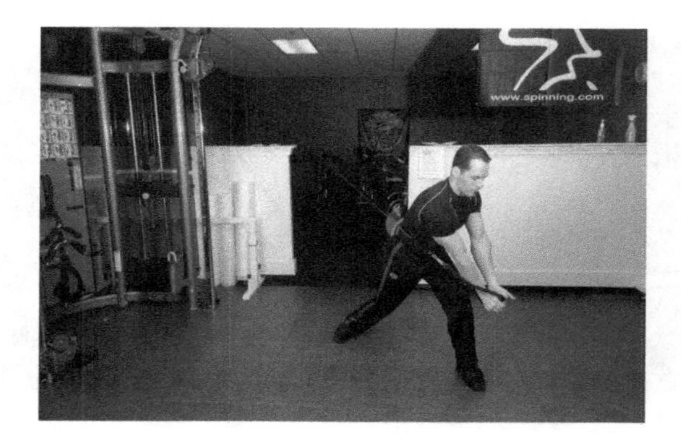


# Start Finish

Set up a high pulley with the handle attachment. Stand in a wide stance. Hold the handle with both hands. The lead hand should be the first hand on the handle, followed by the other hand on top. With hips parallel to the cable turn the torso grabbing hold of the handle. Start with arms extended. You should feel a stretch in the side of the body. Now turn the body through the core, keep the back straight, and slightly lunge. Arms remain straight. Bring the hands over the knee. Keep the chest up and hold position for 1-2 seconds. Return keeping the back straight and arms extended.

# Transverse Cable Rotation

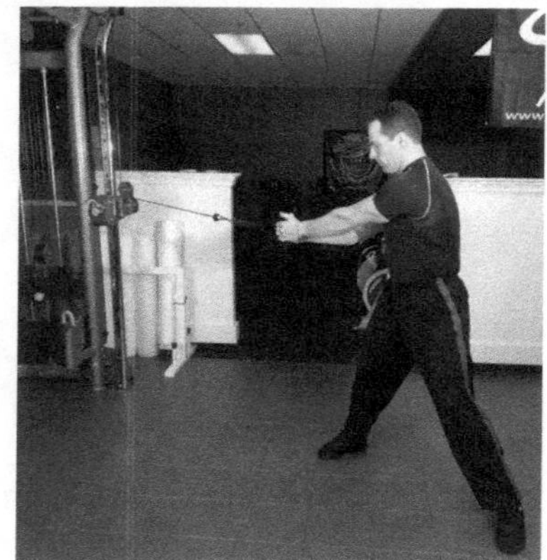

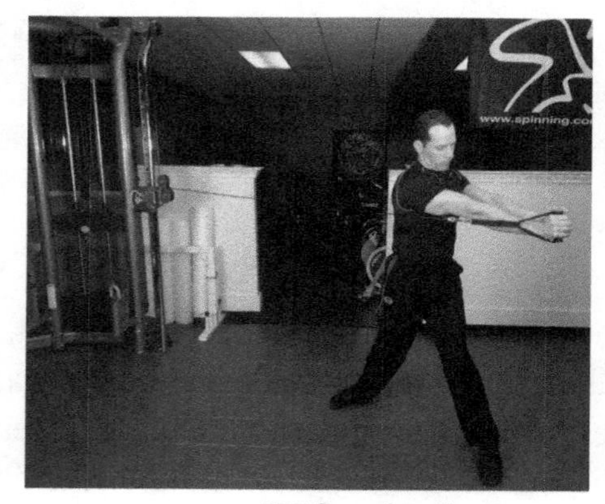

# Start Finish

This exercise is set up the same as the Wood Chop. Rather than performing a downward chopping motion you turn with the hands parallel to the floor. The chest remains up and the back stays straight. You want to focus on turning with the abdominals and not the shoulders. Concentrate on feeing tension in the abdominals, especially the transverse abdominus area. The transverse abdominus is the muscle group that wraps around the body like a belt. It lies underneath the rectus abdominus and internal and external obliques. The transverse abdominus helps support the back during rotational movements.

# Walking Lunges

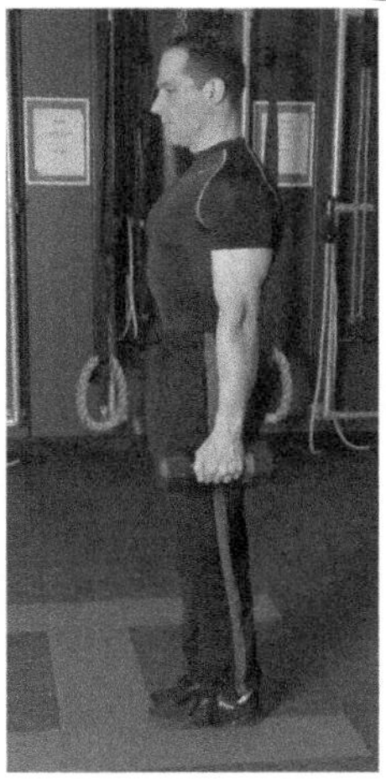

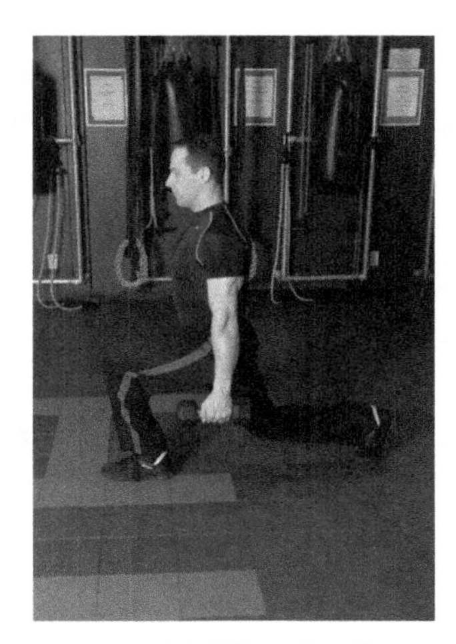

**Start** **Finish**

Stand erect, with dumbells to the side of your body, back straight. Lunge one foot out, drop down so that the leg is at a 80-90 degree position. Keep chest up and back straight. Stand back up. Alternate legs. Do not stay stationary. Perform a moving lunge. Lunging the length of the room and back.

# Lateral Strides w/Dumbell Press

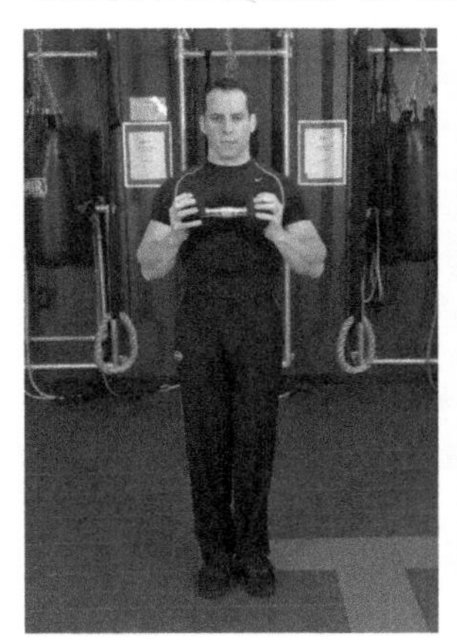

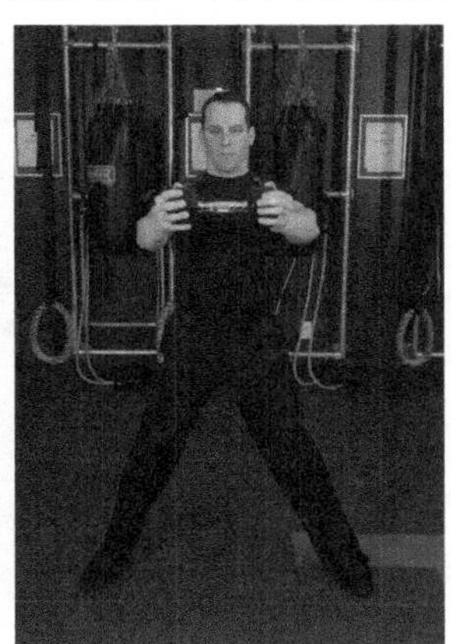

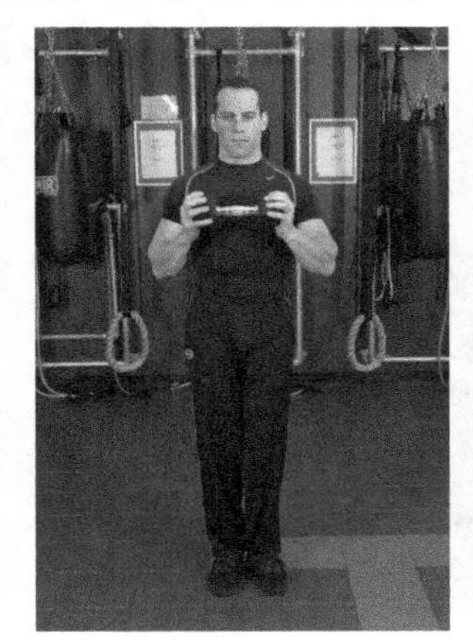

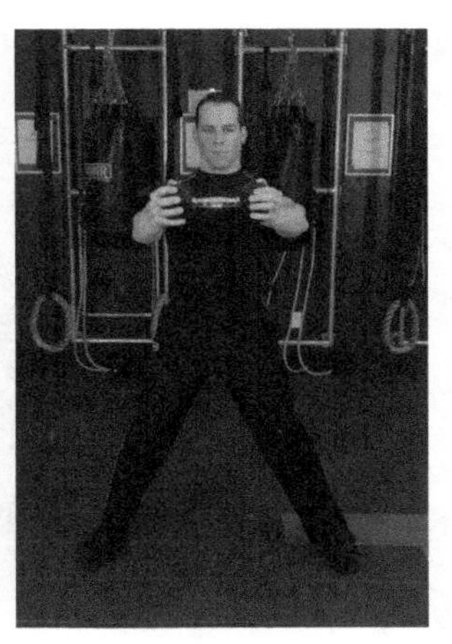

**Start** **Finish**

Start with legs together and holding a dumbell with both hands on the chest. Take a wide side step while simultaneously pushing the dumbell out in front of your chest extending the arms. Bring legs together and bring the dumbell back into the chest. Take another wide step and push the weight out. Continue this pattern moving across the length of the room.

# Medicine Ball Push Ups

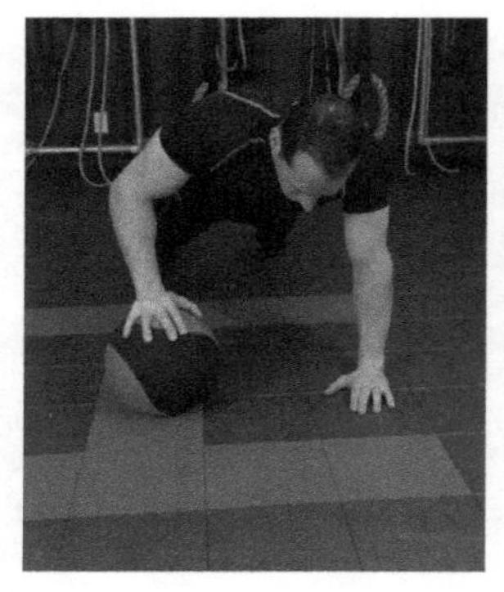
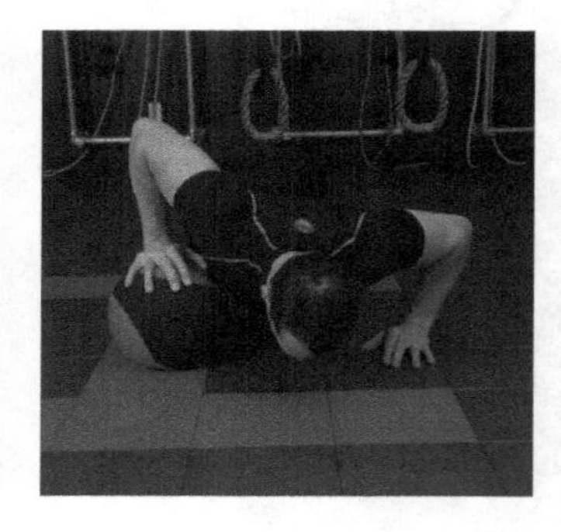
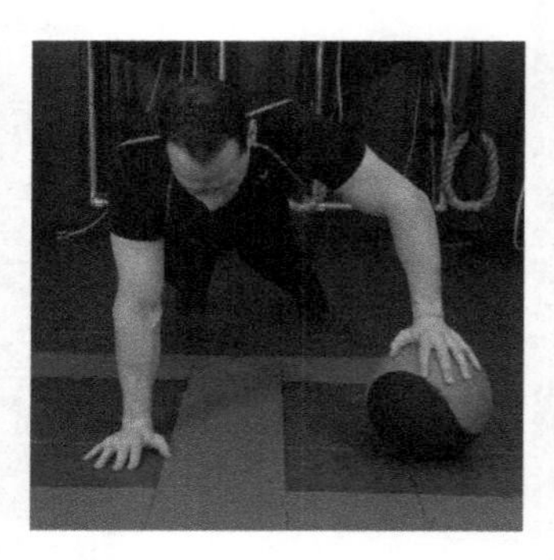

1 2 3

1. Get into a push up position. On your toes, back straight place one hand on a medicine ball with the other hand on the floor.
2. With your hand on the ball drop down bringing the body close to the floor.
3. Push up your body. While back in the extended arm position, roll the ball over to the other hand and perform another push up. Continue rolling the ball back and forth until all repetitions are completed.

# Medicine Up Wood Chop

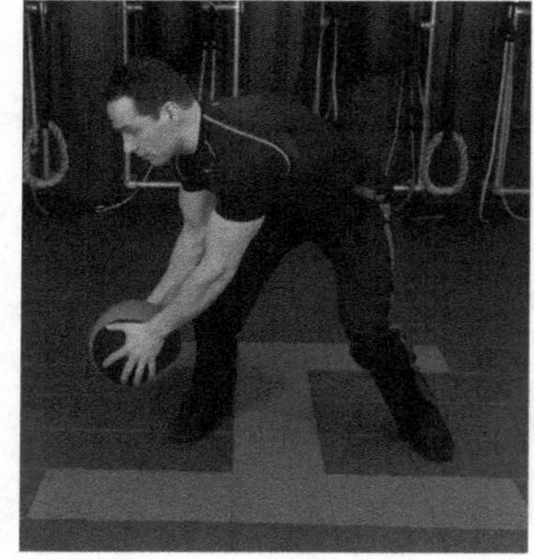
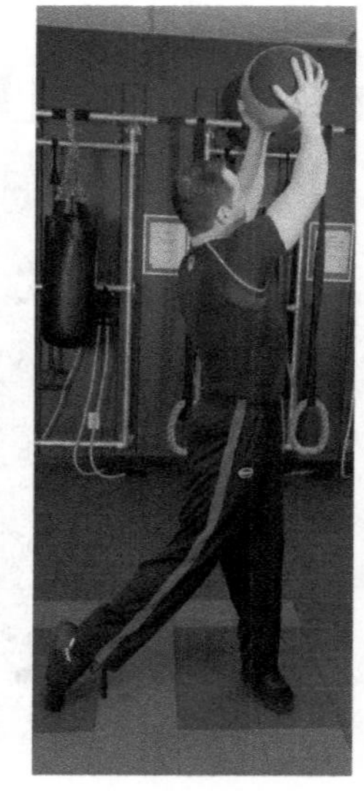

Start Finish

Holding a medicine ball with both hands squat and rotate bringing the ball down close to the outside of the foot. Ascend rotating and across the body, straightening the legs and going up on your toes of the extended leg. Reaching the ball up toward the ceiling, stretch and return to the starting position. Keep the body moving this a dynamic movement and requires core strength and concentration. Many muscles are working to achieve a single task. Start slowly to learn the movement. Progress with more speed when you feel comfortable and strong enough to synchronize the muscle efficiently.

# Exercise: The Metabolic Booster

Exercise is an important part of keeping the body healthy and strong. Many people use exercise as a way to "lose weight." This approach is wrong. As I have discussed losing weight is incorrect and unhealthy. The goal should be to increase lean body tissue and to decrease body fat. Exercise provides a great metabolic boost if performed correctly. The exercise programs that I have outlined are good overall plans to help boost your active metabolism. Keep in mind that the more you exercise the more repair and recovery of damaged muscle tissue is required. To help repair damaged muscle tissue, you need to eat more nutrients than normal. Eating less and exercising more does not make sense. This only perpetuates undesirable muscle loss and fat storage. The more you exercise the more you need eat.

It is important to change up your exercise routine every month. Staying at the same intensity for months will not produce results. It is important to change up the intensity to shock the musculoskeletal and cardiovascular systems of the body. If you would like more exercise programs, I offer an online personal service. For a small fee you can have access to many more programs that will be tailored to match your needs. www.darylconant.com

# Age and Exercise

Everyone can benefit from exercise. There is no age limit. It is important to have a professional help when designing an accurate and safe exercise program. Go to a gym that has a clinical Exercise Physiologist on staff to help with proper exercise prescription. Exercise Physiologist's have an extensive background in cardiac rehabilitation, post-physical therapy rehabilitation, gerontology, kinesiology, exercise physiology, and neural physiology.

Everyone's need vary and when you have a professionally designed plan you can exercise safely and accurately.

People who say that they are too old to exercise are making excuses. There are exercises that everyone can do. Even if an individual is restricted to a wheel chair, they can still exercise and reap the benefits. Weight training is not just for young people. It is very important for older folks as well. In fact, I think it is more important to weight train when we get older because the bone integrity lessens as we age. Weight training can help slow down and possibly regain bone strength and growth. Also, exercising regularly helps develop all the systems of the body.

# The Benefits of Regular Exercise

- Improved digestion
- Enhances quality of sleep
- Improves complexion
- Improves body composition (fat to muscle ratio)
- Makes muscles more forceful
- Greater muscular definition
- Greater fat burning ability
- Increases flexibility
- Improves cardiovascular endurance
- Improves active metabolism
- Improves circulation and helps reduce blood pressure
- Increases lean muscle tissue in the body
- Boost digestive metabolism
- Alleviates menstrual cramps
- Improves clarity, and neural physiology
- Increases metabolic rate
- Enhances coordination and balance
- Improves posture
- Reduces and possibly eliminates back problems and pain
- Lowers resting heart rate
- Increases muscle size through an increase in muscle fibers
- Improves body composition
- Increases body density
- Metabolizes fat and sugar better
- Makes body more agile
- Increases energy
- Reduces joint discomfort
- Improves athletic performance.
- Enriches sexuality /libido.
- Improves overall quality of life
- Increases your range of motion
- Enhances immune system
- Improves glycogen storage
- Enables the body to utilize energy more efficiently
- Increases aerobic and anaerobic enzymes
- Increases the number and size of mitochondria in muscle cells

- Increases concentration of myoglobin (carries oxygen in muscles) in skeletal muscles
- Enhances oxygen transport throughout the body
- Improves liver functions
- Increases speed of muscle contraction and reaction time
- Improves the nervous system neuronal synapse
- Strengthens the heart
- Improves blood flow through arteries and veins
- Helps to alleviate varicose veins
- Increases maximum cardiac output and stroke volume
- Increases contractility of the heart's ventricles
- Increases the weight and size of the heart
- Improves contraction of the heart
- Makes calcium transport in the heart and body more efficient
- Increases sarcoplasmic and sarcomere hypertrophy
- Improves self esteem
- Improves self confidence
- Helps reduce cravings for eating junk food
- Slows down the acquired aging effects
- Builds bone density
- Great stress reducer
- Boosts anabolic hormone levels
- Increased protein metabolism
- Cleansing effect
- Improves immunity
- Anti-depressant
- Increases overall strength
- Helps with anger management
- Repairs and rebuilds muscles from injuries faster
- Improve maximum volume of oxygen levels
- Increases lactate levels
- Increases oxygen saturation levels
- Improves lymphatic system production

# The Set Point Theory: Why We Shouldn't LOSE WEIGHT

From the moment of conception, our DNA coding dictates all cellular processing. Within the DNA are written codes that instruct the cells of how big the muscles will be, how many muscle fibers you will have, how tall you will be, how fast you reproduce cells, and how much fat you should have. Essentially the DNA sets the limits to what your body can and cannot do. If we didn't have these limitations then the body would just keep growing without stopping. Imagine if your body didn't have limits and it was normal for all people to keep growing and growing. There needs to be certain limits to what our body can do. This limit is known as the *set point.*

The set point is the actual weight your body should be at the end of human development. Everyone has a certain set point. For example, I weigh 185 pounds. I have been this weight ever since I was 25. Twenty-five is usually the end point of human body development. Through genetics my DNA is programmed to produce enough bone, muscle, and fat, to maintain a 185 pound body. No matter what I do I will never grow to be six feet 250 pounds. This is impossible. My body is only designed to stay set at 185 pounds, respectively.

Body composition, including fat and muscle ratio, is set in the DNA. As I have discussed in this book, body fat is essential for normal processing of the cells of the body. If you keep your body in the healthy range of body fat and muscle, then that is your correct weight. Whatever your weight is at that point is your set point.

**Here is how you figure your set point weight.**
If you have a body fat percentage of 35% and your weight is 150 pounds, your body is composed of 52.5 pounds of fat and 97.5 of muscle. Your body fat percentage exceeds the healthy norm of the amount of fat a body should have. The healthy range of body fat is, 22-28% for females and 4-22% for men. Clearly having 35% body fat puts you out of your range. By exercising and eating healthy, the body can metabolize off the excess body fat. Now, you are at 24% body fat and weigh 145 pounds. Your total body fat is 34.8 pounds and your muscle equates for 110.2 pounds. The body has been able to adjust by activating more muscle tissue to help burn off the excess fat. This is a good thing. Activating more muscle is the key for changing body composition. This is why it doesn't make sense to me to lose "weight." When you lose weight you lose muscle. So now, whatever your

weight is when you get to a healthy body composition measurement is your set point. In this case the person's set point is roughly 145 pounds. Their DNA is programmed to maintain this number. If you continue to eat poorly and avoid exercising, you alter your set point by storing extra fat and metabolizing off your own muscle tissue.

Social consciousness should be more focused on maintaining healthy body composition values rather than worrying about what the scale says. Forcing your body to drop unnecessary weight compromises your health. The public needs to be more educated on maintaining their set point. We all shouldn't weigh the same weight and all look exactly the same. Everyone has a set point and we should know what it is. That is what being is shape is all about-- healthy body composition ratios.

# Appendix

## I. Dangerous Food Additives and Preservatives - To AVOID!

Do the foods in your cupboards and refrigerator contain any of the following?

***Reaction Symbol: Hyperactivity (H) - Asthma (A) - Cancer (C)***

**Additive or Preservative and Their Reaction**
Acacia Gum (Food Stabilizer) - A
Acetic Acid, Glacial (preservatives) - A
Acid Brilliant Green, Green S, Food Green (food color) H-A
Activated Vegetable Carbons, Brilliant Black (food color) H-A-C
Alkanet (yellow to orange food color) H-C
Allura Red AC (food color) H-A-C
Aluminium (preservatives) - - C
Amaranth (Red food color #2) H-A-C
Annatto Extracts (Food Color) - H-A-C
Anthocyanins Side Effect Unknown
Aspartame (Sweetener) H-A
Azorubine, Carmoisine (food color) H A C
Benzoic Acid (preservatives) H A C
Benzoyl Peroxide (Bleaching Flour and Bread enhancer Agent) - A
Bleached Starch (Thickenner and Stabiliser) - A
Brown FK (Food Color) - H-C
Brilliant Black (Food Color) - C
Brilliant Blue (food color) H A C
Butylated Hydroxyanisole (BHA) (Synthetic Antioxidants) H-A-C
Butylated Hydroxytoluene (BHT) or Butylhydroxytoluene (Synthetic Antioxidants) H A C
Calcium Benzoate (preservatives) - A
Calcium Hydrogen Sulphite (preservatives) - A
Calcium or Potassium or Sodium Propionates, Propionic Acid (preservatives) H A
Calcium Sulphite (preservatives) - A
Camauba Wax (used in Chewing Gums, Coating and Glazing Agents) - - C
Caramel (food color) H
Carmines, Cochineal (food color) H -A
Carrageenan (Thickening & Stabilizing Agent) - A C
Chlorine (Agent used in Bleaching Flour, Bread Enhancer and Stabilizer) - - C

Chlorine Dioxide (Bleaching Flour and Preservative Agent) - - C
Chocolate Brown HT, Brown HT (food color) H A
CDiphenyl, Biphenyl (preservatives) - - C
Citrus Red No. 2 (Red Food Color - C
Cyclamate and Cyclamic Acid (Sweeteners) - - C
Disodium Guanylate (Flavor Enhancers) H A
Disodium Inosinate 5 (Flavor Enhancers) - A
Disodium Ribonucleotides 5 (Flavor Enhancers) - A
Dodecyl Gallate (Synthetic Antioxidant) - A -
Ethyl Para Hydroxybenzonate (preservatives) - A
Erythrosine (Red food color #2) H A C
Fast Green (food color) - A -H
Fast Yellow AB (A synthetically manufactured azo dye - C
Food Brown, Kipper Brown, Brown FK (food color) H A C
Formaidehyde (Preservative) - C
Formic Acid (preservative) - - C
Gardenia Yellow (Food Color) Side Effects Unknown
Gelatine (Food Gelling Agent) - A
Glycerol (Sweetener, Bulking Agent) - Coverts into Fat
Guanylic Acid 5 (Flavor Enhancer) H-A-C
Hexamine, Hexamethylene Tetramine (preservatives) - - C
Hydrochloric Acid (Hydrolyzing Enhancer & Gelatin Production) - - C
Indigotine, Indigo Carmine (food color) H A C
Insoluble Polyvinylpyrrolidone Insoluble (Stabilizer and Clarifying Agent added to Wine, Beer, Pharmaceuticals) - - C
Latol Rubine, Pigment Rubine (preservatives) H A C
Lycopenes - C
Karaya Gum (Laxative, Food Thickener & Emulsifier) - A
Magnesium Sulphate (Tofu Coagulant) - - C
Manascorubin (Food Color Blue RS) -H-A-C-
Mannitol (Artificial Sweetener) H -
MSG Monosodium Glutamate, Glutamic Acid, all Glutamates H A C
Methyl p-Hydroxybenzoate (Preservative) -C
Norbixin, Annatto Extracts (yellow, red to brown natural colors) H- A
Orthophenyl Phenol (preservatives) - - C
Octyl Gallate (Synthetic Antioxidant) - A
Paraffin, Vaseline, White Mineral Oil (Solvents, Coating, Glazing, Anti Foaming, Lubricant Agents in Chewing Gums) - - C
Patent Blue (food color) H-A-C
Pectins (Thickener) - C

Propyl p-Hydroxybenzoate (Preservative) -C
Ponceau, Brilliant Scarlet (food color) H A C
Polysorbate (Emulsifiers) - - C
Polyxyl Stearate (Emulsifier) - - C
Polyoxyethylene Sorbitan Monostearate (Emulsifiers Gelling Stabilisers Thickeners Agents) - - C
Polyxyethylene Stearate (Emulsifier) - - C
Potassium Bromate (Agent used in Bleaching Flour) - - C
Potassium & Calcium Sorbates ,Sorbic Acid (preservatives) H A
Propyl Gallate (Synthetic Antioxidant) - A C
Propyl P Hydroxybenzonate, Propylparaben (preservatives) - A
Potassium Acesulphame (Sweetener) - - C
Potassium Bisulphite, Potassium Hydrogen Sulphite (preservatives) H- A
Potassium Ferrocyanide (Anti Caking Agent) - A
Potassium Metabisulfite (preservatives) - A
Potassium Nitrate (preservative) - A C
Potassium Sulfite (preservatives) - A
Quinoline Yellow (food color) H A C
Red 2G (Red food color) H A C
Saccharine (Sweetener) - - C
Sodium Benzoate (preservatives) H A
Sodium Bisulphite (preservatives) - A
Sodium CarboxyMethyl Cellulose - - C
Sodium Ethyl Para Hydroxybenzonate (preservatives) - A
Sodium Hydrogen Sulphite (Preservative) - C
Sodium Metabisulphite (preservatives) - A
Sodium Nitrate (preservative) H - C
Sodium Nitrite (preservative) H A C Sodium Propyl P Hydroxybenzonate (preservatives) - A
Sodium Sulphite (preservatives) - A
Sorbic Acid (Preservative) - C
Sorbitol & Sorbital Syrup - (Sweetener, Bulking Agent) H
Sulphur Dioxide (preservatives) H A -
Sunset Yellow (Yellow food color #6) H A C
Talc (Anti Caking, Filling, Softener, Agent) - - C
Tartrazine (food color) H A C
TBHQ, Tert Butylhydroquinone (Synthetic Antioxidants) H A -
Titanium Dioxide (Food Color) Side Effects Unknown
Tragacanth (thickener & Emulsifier) - A -
Yellow 2G (food color) H A C

**These are only some of the dangers that lurk in our food supply. I suggest that you become a food detective and read as much as you can about the poisons that are in our food supply. You will be shocked at how many toxic chemicals are used to preserve food. As I said earlier, there is direct link between these toxic chemicals and illness. I am a firm believer that most cancers, illness, and disease can be reduced if our food supply were to become natural and toxin free.**

# II. Modern Day Supplements

## Please Note:

***There are many different supplements that are on the market, too many to write about. I have chosen the most common ones that many Americans take on a daily basis. This list is just a helpful guide for knowing the different types of supplements and their dosages. It is important to do research and/or see a doctor before taking supplements.**

## Supplements for Daily Nutrition/ General Health / Improve Immunity

**4- Androstenediol:** Anabolic agent. Anti-catabolic. Recommended dose 300-600 mg daily

**19-Norandrostenediol:** Anabolic agent. Anti-catabolic. Recommended dose 300-600 mg daily.

**19-Norandrostenedione:** Anabolic agent. Anti-catabolic. Recommended dose 300-600 mg daily.

**Alanine:** Promotes facilitation of glucose production. Prevents muscle breakdown. Recommended dose 1-3 g daily.

**Alpha-ketoglutarate (AKG):** Helps prevent muscle breakdown. Enhances oxygen delivery. Recommended dose 3-4

**Androstenedione:** Anabolic agent. Anti-catabolic. Recommended dose 50-100 mg daily.

**Arabinogalactin:** helps boost immunity and fights against infections. Recommended dose 1.5-3 g daily.

**Arginine:** Promotes growth hormone release. Immune system enhancer. Improves blood flow in male genitals. Recommended dose 5-15 g daily.

**Arginine Ketoisocaproate (AKC):** Helps boost brain activity. Prevent muscle breakdown. Recommended Dose: 4-6 g daily.

**Beta-ecdysterone:** Balances nitrogen levels. Recommended dose 1-1.5 g daily.

**Beta-glucan:** helps boost immunity and fights against infections. Recommended dose. 3-6 g daily.

**B-hydroxy-B methylbutyrate (HMB):** Prevents muscle breakdown. Recommended dose. 3-5 g daily

**Branched Chain Amino Acids:** Helps rebuild muscle tissue. Recommended dose 5-10 g daily.

**Choline:** Helps with muscle contraction. Lipotropic agent. Helps nourish nerves and membranes. Recommended dose 500 mg - 1g daily.

**Chondroitin Sulfate:** Joint health and anti-inflammatory support. Recommended dose. 1.2-1.5 g daily.

**Chrysin:** Anti-estrogen agent. 1-3 g daily.

**Colostrum:** Substance found in mother's breast milk. Immune enhancer. Recommended dose. 150-2 g daily.

**Conjugated Linoleic Acid (CLA):** Lipotropic agent. Helps increase lean body mass. Decreases body fat. Recommended dose 2-4 daily.

**Copper:** Aids in joint health. Recommended dose. 1.5 mg daily.

**Creatine:** Increases cellular creatine phosphate levels to bind with adenosine diphosphate to produce ATP. Buffers ATP/CP system for longer duration of power and strength. Cell volumizer. Recommended dose 2-20 g daily.

**D-Ribose:** Regulate sugar metabolism, ergogenic aid. Improve recovery. Recommended dose 2.5-5 g daily.

**Dehydroepiandrosterone (DHEA):** Increases testosterone levels. Recommended dose 25-100 mg daily.

**DL- Phenylalanine:** Pain reliever. Recommended dose. 250-500 mg daily.

**Glutamine:** Help prevents muscle breakdown. Immune system. Recommended dose 5-20 g daily.

**Glycerol:** Helps maintain plasma volume. Helps hydration. Recommended dose 6-8 g daily.

**Ipriflavone:** Promotes lean body mass. Can help improve bone strength. Recommended dose 600 mg daily.

**Ketoisocaproic acid/ketoisocaproate:** Prevents muscle breakdown. Recommended dose 4-6 g daily.

**Medium-chain triglycerides (MCT):** Improves energy. Lipotropic agent. Recommended dose 8-20 g daily.

**Methoxyisoflavone:** Increases lean body mass. Recommended dose 500mg -1 g daily.

**Ornithine:** Promotes growth hormone release. Prevents muscle breakdown. Recommended dose 5-10 g daily.

**Ornithine-alpha-ketoglutarate (OKG):** Hormone precursor. Helps prevent muscle breakdown. Recommended dose 6-8 g daily.

**Phosphatidyserine (PS):** Improve mental acuity. Lowers cortisol levels. Recommended dose 200-800 mg daily.

**Pregnenolone:** Anabolic agent. Increases testosterone. Recommended dose 100-200 mg daily.

**Taurine:** Cell volumizer. Anti-catabolic. Anti-oxidant. Recommended dose 1-3 g daily.

**Tribulus Terrestris:** Anabolic agent. Improves erection in men. Improves strength. Recommended dose 750 mg-1.5 g daily.

**ZMA (Zinc monomethionine aspartate, magnesium aspartate, B6):** Maintain testosterone and IGF-1 levels; helps improve strength. Can improve sleep/recovery. Recommended dose 2-3 capsules daily. Recommended dose 2-3 capsules daily.

## Supplements for Weight Loss. Improved Energy and Endurance.

**Acetyl-L Carnitine:** Testosterone enhancer. Can lower cholesterol. Improve mental acuity. Recommended dose 500-750 mg daily.

**Alpha-lipoic Acid (ALA):** Antioxidant. Improves cholesterol levels. Recommended dose 200-800 mg daily.

**Chromium:** Helps maintain glucose metabolism. Increases lean body mass. Recommended dose 100-400 mcg daily.

**Co-enzyme Q10:** Antioxidant clearing free radicals out of blood. Improves energy production. Heart health Recommended dose 100-400 mg daily.

**Colosolic Acid:** Helps regulate blood glucose.

**Conjugated Linoleic Acid (CLA):** Lipotropic agent. Helps increase lean body mass, decreases body fat. Recommended dose 2-4 daily.

**Goat Weed:** Improves sexual performance. Increases endurance. Improves energy. Recommended dose 500 mg-2 g daily.

**Guggulsterones:** Provides thyroid support. Reduces cholesterol. Recommended dose 200-800 mg daily.

**Hydroxy Citric Acid (HCA):** Prevents sugar from turning into fat. Appetite suppressant.

**L-Carnitine:** Increases fatty acid delivery to muscle cells. Increases endurance. Recommended dose 2-4 g daily.

**Pyruvate:** Helps decrease body fat. Improves energy. Recommended dose 5-10 g daily.

**Sodium Bicarbonate:** Helps improve anaerobic metabolism. Recommended dose 300mg/kg 1-3 hours before exercise.

**Yohimbine:** Male libido enhancer. Thermogenic aid. Recommended dose 15-20 mg daily.

## Supplements for General Health and Conditioning.

**Charcoal:** Liver cleanser. Immune booster. Recommended dose 5g daily.

**DL-Phenylalanine:** Pain inhibitor. Recommended dose 250-500 mg daily.

**Echinacea:** Helps fight against colds. Immune booster. Recommended dose 500-1 g daily.

**Essential Fatty Acids (DHA and EPA):** Lipotropic agents to help nourish the cells of the body. Recommended dose 2-30 g daily.

**Flaxseed Oil:** Great source of EFA's. Improves cardiovascular health. Anti-carcinogenic agent. Recommended dose 2 Tbsp. Or 2-4 capsules daily.

**Glucosamine:** Joint anti-inflammatory. Has been known to reduce connective tissue pain. Recommended dose 1.5-3 g daily.

**Goldenseal:** Helps fight against colds. Immune booster. Recommended dose 250-750 g daily.

**Green Tea:** Antioxidant. Fights against free radicals. Promotes relaxation. Boosts metabolism. Recommended dose 1-2 cups daily.

**L-Histidine:** Anti-inflammatory agent.

**L-Lysine:** An essential amino acid. Helpful in reduction of herpes virus, cold sores. Can help bone growth and skin health. Recommended dose 500 mg- 1 g daily.

**N-Acetylcysteine (NAC):** Immune booster and antioxidant. Recommended dose 1-1.5 g daily.

**Olive Leaf Extract:** Immune system enhancer. Helps fight against infections. Recommended dose 500mg-2 g daily.

**Primrose Oil:** Inflammatory agent. Can reduce arthritic pain and swelling. Can help alleviate PMS symptoms. Recommended dose 500 mg daily.

**Protein Powders: (Including casein, whey, egg, soy protein):** Ample supply of amino acids, vitamins and minerals to nourish the body. Recommended dose 20-200 g daily.

**Psyllium Seed:** Promotes regularity in bowels, immunity and cleansing effect in intestines. Recommended dose 1 tbsp. daily

**Saw Palmetto:** Nourishes prostate gland. Anti-dihydrostesterone. Recommended dose 200-350 mg daily.

## Supplements for Weight Loss

**Alpha-lipoic Acid (ALA):** Antioxidant. Improves cholesterol levels. Recommended dose 200-800 mg daily.

**Chromium Picolinate:** Aids in glucose metabolism. Increases the efficiency of insulin production. Recommended dose 100-400 mg daily.

**Co-Enzyme Q10:** Antioxidant clearing free radicals out of blood. Improves energy production. Heart health Recommended dose 100-400 mg daily.

**Conjugated Linoleic Acid (CLA):** Lipotropic agent. Anticarcinogenic.

**Flaxseed Oil:** Great source of EFA's. Improves cardiovascular health. Anti-carcinogenic agent. Recommended dose 2 Tbsp. Or 2-4 capsules daily.

**L-Carnitine:** Increases fatty acid delivery to muscle cells. Increases endurance. Recommended dose 2-4 g daily.

## Supplements for Psychological Balance

**5-HTP (5-hydroxytryptophan):** Stress reducer; Promotes sleep state. Recommended dose 50-100 mg daily.

**Acetyl-L Carnitine:** Testosterone enhancer. Can lower cholesterol. Improve mental acuity. Recommended dose 500-750 mg daily.

**Choline:** Improve structure of cell membranes, helps protect liver from over production of fat. Is a precursor molecule for the neurotransmitter acetylcholine. Recommended dose 500 mg- 1 g daily.

**Kava-kava:** Anti-anxiety agent. Promotes relaxation. Recommended dose 45-70 mg daily.

**Ginko Biloba:** Improves brain oxygen flow. Improves mental concentration. Recommended dose 80-100 mg daily.

**L-Theanine:** Creates a sense of relaxation stimulates the production of alpha brain waves, creating a state of deep relaxation and mental alertness. Involved in the formation of the inhibitory neurotransmitter, gamma amino butyric acid (GABA). GABA influences dopamine and serotonin, producing relaxation. Recommended dose 200 mg-1 g daily.

**Melatonin:** Helps sleep patterns. Immune booster. Recommended dose 1-3 capsules before bed.

**SAMe (S-adenosyl-l-methionine):** Osteoarthritis, depression, liver disease. Recommended dose 400 mg daily.

**St. John's Wart:** Anti-depressant. Mood enhancer. Recommended dose 750 mg- 1 g daily.

**Tyrosine:** Building block for serotonin, norepinephrine, epinephrine. Mood enhancer. 2-3 g daily.

**Valerian Root:** Reduces stress, anxiety, and nervousness. Recommended dose 150-300 mg daily.

# III. Boosting Your Active Metabolism

As discussed earlier, the resting metabolic rate is the amount of energy that the body expends to maintain the VNES. It is the absolute minimal energy requirement for the body to live. When we move around doing normal human activities we are increasing our metabolic processes. This is known as *active metabolism.* By increasing the active metabolism, the thermogenic effect will last longer allowing fat to be burned up more efficiently.

Exercise is the most efficient and quickest way to boost the active metabolism. Looking great and maintaining the correct ratio of fat and lean body mass depends on proper nutrition and exercise techniques. I believe that having a great looking physique is eighty-five percent nutrition and fifteen percent exercise. Here are some myths about exercise that are common among fitness enthusiasts.

**Myth: I Will Lose Weight If I Exercise More and Eat Less?**

The idea of exercising more and eating less is misleading. People that have no prior experience with exercising or a comprehensive knowledge of how their metabolism works usually fall into an unbalanced regime. Exercising too much and not taking in the correct amount of nutrients to supply the VNES will result in catabolic metabolism.

**Fact:**
The more you exercise the more nutrients you need to take in. The VNES must be fed to sustain human life. When you exercise, more nutrients are being consumed by active organs to keep up with the demand of the muscles. By cutting down your external nutrient intake you won't be able to supply the body with the accurate amount of nutrients to feed the VNES. The result is you will lose weight, but mostly muscle tissue. The fat cells won't release fat because the body will be in catabolic metabolism. Losing lean body mass is not a desirable effect.

Example: Jane 175 pounds 35 years old, 30% body fat, resting metabolic rate 1500 vital nutrient calories. She wants to lose 25 pounds.

Jane came to me for help. She wanted to lose twenty-five pounds. When I asked her how she came up with twenty-five pounds she told me that she just thinks that she will look better if she lost twenty-five pounds. There was really no reason or explanation for losing that much weight. I then asked her how she intended to lose the weight. She told me that, "everyone tells me that you have to exercise on the treadmill for forty-five minutes to two hours and eat only one to two times a day. I eat one egg for breakfast, a container of yogurt for lunch and a salad for dinner. By cutting down on my eating I assume I will lose weight faster." This type of thinking is how most Americans think when it comes to losing weight. This way of thinking will only promote catabolic metabolism. Fat will not be burned but muscle will. I told Jane that if she continued to follow her plan that she would lose weight but it would be mostly muscle. Unfortunately, she didn't want to listen to my advice and she decided to continue on her plan. Here are the results.

Before:
Exercise: 90 Minutes Treadmill. 30 minutes weight training.
Weight 175
Body Fat: 30%

- 52.5 pounds total fat
- 122.5 pounds total lean body mass (muscle, bone, tissue)

After (4 Months)
Weight 160
Body Fat: 33%

- 52.8 pounds total fat
- 107.2 pounds total lean body mass (muscle, bone, water)

Total: No loss in fat weight. Loss in lean body mass 15.3 pounds. She lost weight but now has less muscle. Her body has been in catabolic metabolism.

The goal should have been to increase the lean body mass activity to help metabolize off the excess fat. When I explained to her the disadvantages of losing muscle rather than fat, she finally changed her way of thinking and began to follow my advice. Here is what she did. I had her follow a nutrient dense nutritional plan and prescribed an effective exercise program.

Exercise: Circuit Training: 30 minutes
Nutrient Intake: 5-6 small, nutrient dense meals per day.

The result four months later.

Weight 150 (which is the ideal weight for her)
Body Fat: 24%

- 36 pounds total fat

*Continued*

-114 pounds total lean body mass (muscle, bone, water)

She lost 16.8 pounds of fat and gained back 7 pounds of lean body mass. The activation of lean body mass shows that her body is maintaining anabolic metabolism. By losing the 16.8 pounds of fat her physical appearance had significantly changed. She looked more defined and healthy.

**Myth: Weighing yourself on a scale is a good way to measure fitness.**

False.

**Fact:**

Scales should only be used for medical purposes to determine if a person is losing or gaining weight drastically during disease or illness. This information is useful for doctors to determine the validity of drug and nutrition therapy. However, scales are useless for determining your fitness level. Many people become obsessed with weighing themselves. It is amazing, but the scale can actually make or break a person's personality for the day. If the person gets on the scale and the number is lower than the day before, they will be happy and feel better about themselves. They will go to work feeling lighter and more confident. If the person gets on the scale and the number is higher than the day before, they will become angry, depressed, sad, and/or dejected. They will go to work feeling withdrawn and overly obsessed with thoughts of being fat.

People feel that in order to feel good about themselves and to be classified as being fit that they have to weigh a certain amount. This is just ridiculous! Losing weight for the sake of losing weight is ignorant thinking. When I talk to clients about changing how they look and feel I always refer to LOSING FAT not WEIGHT. However, when I mention losing weight, I sell more programs than I do if I mention losing fat weight. Which leads me to believe that many people have not been properly educated on body composition.

Body composition is broken down into two parts, body fat and lean body mass.

Body fat consists of subcutaneous fat, inter and intramuscular fat, and visceral fat. Subcutaneous fat, is the fat (adipose) underneath the skin covering the musculoskeletal system. Subcutaneous is needed to help insulate the body and provides protection.

Inter muscular fat is fat that is stored outside in between muscle cells.
Inter muscular fat is available for fueling the muscles to produce energy for the body. Intra muscular fat is the fat that is inside the muscle cell. Intra muscular fat provides fat soluble vitamins and energy to working muscle tissue.

Visceral fat is the fat that collects and stores around the vital organs of in the visceral region. The stomach, omentum, intestines, liver, kidneys, spleen, gallbladder, and pancreas all comprise the visceral region. Though visceral fat is important for proper nourishment, nourishment, insulation, and protection of the vital organs, if too much visceral fat is present, the risk of developing cardiovascular disease and digestive disease increases. The human body can withstand large amounts of fat storage subcutaneously and inter muscularly without putting too much strain on the heart. The heart has to work harder if the body has too much visceral fat. This is because the visceral fat bogs down the functioning of the other vital organs.

The human body has to have a certain amount of fat to maintain healthy functioning.

For men 4-18% of body fat is considered normal and healthy. Fat percentages beyond 18% can begin compromise the health of vital organs. Body fat percentages 19-24% is considered Over Weight. Body fat percentages 25-30% is considered Obese. Body fat percentages 31+ is considered Morbidly Obese.

For women 18-28% of body fat is considered normal and healthy. Fat percentages beyond 28% can begin to compromise the health of vital organs. Body fat percentages 29-31% is considered Over Weight. Body fat percentages 32-35% is considered Obese. Body fat percentages 35+ is considered Morbidly Obese.

***Understanding Your Ideal weight.***
We all have a set weight that is programmed in our DNA (Deoxyribonucleic acid). The DNA is the genetic coding of our existence. The DNA determines height, weight, cellular production, tissue size, etc. Everyone has a different DNA code. We all have a predetermined body weight. Body weight is determined by how many cells your body needs to maintain the DNA coding. The DNA has a set code for the amount of fat and Lean Body Mass a person should have. If you maintain a healthy fat percentage then whatever your weight is that at that point is considered your ideal weight. The goal is to maintain health fat percentages. Don't worry about weight. You should only be concerned with body fat percentages. Your DNA has determined your weight and as long as you stay within the healthy percentages

of body fat then weight doesn't matter. It is dangerous to lose weight just to get to a specific arbitrary number. It is all about maintaining a healthy body fat percentage to muscle percentage NOT WEIGHT.

Mentally Americans are too fixated on the "losing weight."
It is interesting to me when I advertise my programs in the newspaper. I will put in the ad Daryl Conant's Fat Loss System. Thinking that fat loss will be the hook to get people into the program. However, I don't get any response to the ad. When I put an ad in that reads Daryl Conant's Weight Loss System, I get a tremendous response and new sign ups. People need to be better educated about losing body fat, and understand that just losing "weight" is not an accurate goal.

**Myth: Lifting weights will turn women into muscle bound men.**

Women fear that if they lift weights that they will become muscle bound like a male body builder. They will resort to doing countless hours of cardiovascular exercise to lose body fat instead of lifting weights.

**Fact:**
Weight training will not make you look muscle bound like a bodybuilder unless you train specifically for that effect. Regular resistance training provides great benefits. Increased bone density, immunity boost, fat metabolism, increased lean body mass activity are all benefits of resistance training. To develop muscle like a body builder it takes a tremendous amount of discipline, genetics and hormonal support. A person has to be disciplined to proper nutritional support, supplement and training schedules to increase muscle tissue beyond their natural DNA make up. Most women cannot develop hard dense muscle like a male bodybuilder unless they take anabolic agents.

In order to maximize fat burning, weight training is essential. In order to get the most out your muscle tissue it is important to increase its activity. Dormant muscle cells do not burn fat. The more muscle tissue you can activate, the more fat you can burn, and that is the truth!

**Myth: Cardiovascular exercise is the best method for metabolizing fat from the body.**

Many people believe that if they walk or run on treadmill for hours they will lose tons of body fat. Though there are benefits from performing cardiovascular exercise, it is not the best for burning overall fat. The greatest fat burner of all is resistance training.

Cardiovascular (aerobic) exercise is good for developing the cardio-respiratory system (heart and lungs). When you perform aerobic exercise you work at different heart rate intensities. Over time the body will adapt to the cardiovascular exercise to maintain the activity. The body becomes more fit by adapting to the different levels of stress. When adaptation occurs, the body is more efficient at conserving energy. Fat and sugar metabolism is regulated better in fit individuals as opposed to unfit people. The unfit person will burn more calories at first. As they become more fit they will burn fewer calories because their body systems have improved and have become more efficient. After a while the person won't see any significant changes in their body composition. In order to see changes in body composition, it is important to incorporate resistance training. Once you complete the exercise session the body gets back down to the resting metabolic rate quickly and any residual fat burning ceases.

Resistance training (weight training) utilizes sugar as the primary fuel. If the right intensities are used during weight training the muscle will use up its stored sugar. You can feel this happen during the exercise when you feel the pain. The pain in the muscle is when lactic acid is building up in the muscle. Lactic acid is a product of sugar metabolism within the muscle. After you are done performing resistance training the body transfers from sugar metabolism to fat metabolism. The muscles remain hot after resistance training. This is known as the thermogenic effect. This thermogenic effect can last between 30 minutes-6 hours after weight training. During this time fat is being metabolized. How long the residual fat burning effect lasts depends on the intensity of the weight training session.

If you want to burn the most fat and increase lean body mass activity--weight train.

# What to Eat Before and After Exercising

**Before Exercise**

Nutrients are important to provide the body with energy before exercise. It is important to eat a balanced meal with protein and low glycemic carbohydrates one to two hours before exercising. For example; a cup of cottage cheese, or a protein shake, or steak and spinach, or chicken and a small salad, or one tablespoon of almond butter on a piece of seven to twelve grain bread.

Exercising on an empty stomach can to lead low blood sugar and nausea. When the body's sympathetic nervous system is activated sugar levels deplete, while norepinephrine and adrenaline increase. Too much adrenaline in the stomach can cause feelings of nausea. When sugar levels drop and the blood pressure is high this reduces oxygen flow to the brain and causes an individual to feel dizzy or lightheaded.

Avoid eating simple sugars or refined sugars before working out. Orange juice, sports drinks, bananas, candy, cookies, and other high glycemic foods will cause a drop in blood sugar levels. Exercising after ingesting these types of foods can leave you feeling ill.

**Ultra Endurance Activity**

If you are a long distance runner or cyclist it is recommended that you consume low glycemic foods to sustain proper glycogen levels in the muscle. For example, eating one to two cups of wheat pasta two to three hours before the event, or eating peanut butter on whole wheat bread, or a baked potato with one tablespoon of sour cream can be consumed to provide the muscles with enough glycogen to last for up to one to three hours.

**What to Consume During Exercise**

The most important fluid to drink is water. It is important to sip water during the workout to keep the body hydrated. Avoid drinking large quantities of water during exercise. Excessive amounts of water can cause cramping and stir up too much stomach acid resulting in heart burn. Drinking too much water can cool the body down too fast causing a shift in blood from the extremities. This can cause dizziness or ill feelings. It is best to sip water from a water bottle and not a water fountain. When drinking from a water fountain more air than water is consumed. Too much air in the stomach can cause bloating or indigestion.

Sports drinks, in my opinion, are overrated. If taken properly they can help maintain blood sugar levels. Drinking a sports drink before exercise when the muscles are not in need of sugar, will cause a drop in blood sugar levels.

When the muscles are warmed up and some muscle sugar has been depleted, sipping a glucose polymer or a crystalline fructose sport drink can be useful i.e,. Vitamin Water™. Avoid drinking heavy corn syrup and sucrose drinks. These types of drinks can make you feel sluggish.

**Lipotropic Agent**
To increase the transportation of fatty acids into the muscle cell for oxidation, taking the amino acid L-Carnitine 30 minutes to 1 hour prior to exercise can help. L-Carnitine is an essential amino acid that binds with fatty acids to be delivered into the muscle to get metabolized. A tablespoon of liquid L-Carnitine can be diluted with water and sipped during the workout to help boost the fat burning process.

**What to Consume After Exercise**
As discussed earlier in this book, exercise, is a metabolic booster. One of the goals of exercise is to increase the temperature of the muscles (thermogenic effect) to become more permeable for burning fat and sugar. To take advantage of the permeability of muscle tissue and to replenish the muscle with protein, fat, and sugar, eating within 30 minutes to an hour after an exercise session is necessary. Eating a nutrient dense meal balanced with concentrated protein, essential fats and low glycemic carbohydrates is the best. Consuming a protein shake with flaxseed oil or safflower oil in raw organic milk is a good choice to feed tired muscles. An egg omelette with spinach and cheddar cheese is also a good meal to have. The important factor to remember, is that you need to consume a balanced meal within the thermogenic process to get the best result. To stop the catabolic effect as fast as possible is the idea.

# IV. Supplement Distributors

**Natural Source Products**
**Owner: Ron Kosloff**
**Detroit, Michigan**
**1-313-372-1807**

**Raw Indulgence, LTD**
**923 Saw Mill River Rd**
**Ardsley, NY**
**1-866-498-4671**

**The Fitness Nut House**
**Owner: Daryl Conant, M.Ed**
**45 Portland Road**
**Kennebunk, Maine 04043**

**www.thefitnessnut.com**
**www.darylconant.com**
**email: dconant2004@yahoo.com**
**email: fitnessnuthouse@gmail.com**

## Disclaimer

The information provided in this book is not intended to treat, diagnose, or cure illness or disease. Check with your primary care physician before changing or starting a new nutrition plan based on the information in this book. If you have any questions regarding the information in this book, please feel free to contact me.

*--Daryl*

# About the Author

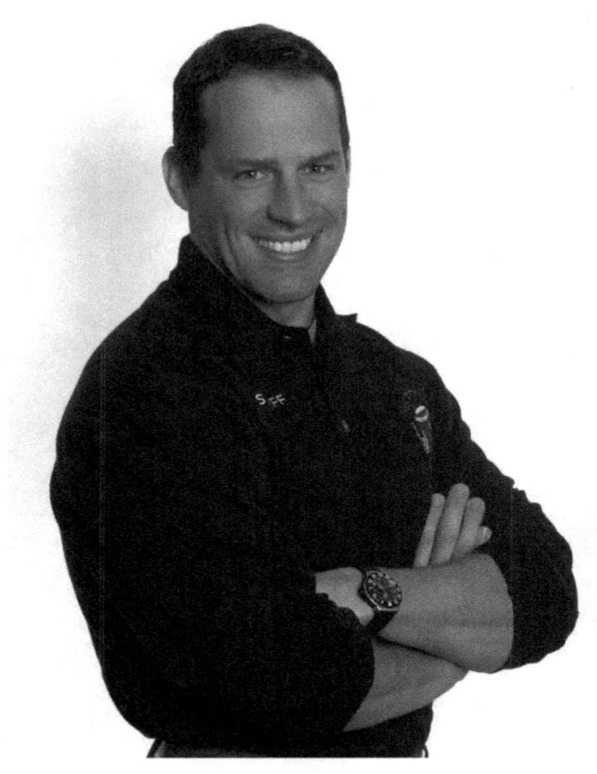

Daryl Conant, Exercise Physiologist and owner of Fitness Nut Enterprises, LLC in Kennebunk, Maine is one of the most sought after fitness figures in the industry today has devoted his life to the pursuit of fitness and nutrition. Over the past twenty years, Daryl has taught thousands of people how to exercise and eat correctly. His insight into exercise and nutrition is both intelligent and motivating. Daryl wrote diet Earth to help people gain control of their life through better eating and exercise methods.

*If humans continue to be unaware of the poisons that are in our food and depend on processed, chemical ladened food for nutrition, obesity, cancer, psychological disorders will continue to prevail.*

*It is time to take a stand and to fight for the right to eat REAL, natural food, free from pesticides, antibiotics, steroids, undigestible poisons, chemical and exocitotoxins. The TRUE health care system is teaching people how to eat healthy and exercise properly; it is not about pumping people up with drugs to live.*

*I hope that Diet Earth has helped you gain a better understanding of how the body works and what you can do to create a healthy practical nutrition plan. I have learned a tremendous amount of information about nutrition over the years and am continuing to learn more. This is not the end all be all to nutrition books. It is my contribution and it is what I believe to be a helpful resource of information about how to eat, why we eat, when to eat, and what to eat. I challenge you to learn as much as possible about the food that you eat, so that you too can become more conscious about the Earth's vital nutrients and their importance in keeping the human body healthy.*

*Thank you for your support*
*Daryl Conant, M.Ed 2010*

CPSIA information can be obtained
at www.ICGtesting.com
Printed in the USA
FSHW02n1101020818
51104FS

9 781452 014371